Clinical Sedation in Dentistry

Clinical Sedation in Dentistry

Written by

Professor N. M. Girdler
Newcastle University Dental School

Mr C. M. Hill
University Dental Hospital, Cardiff

Dr K. E. Wilson
Newcastle Dental Hospital

WILEY-BLACKWELL
A John Wiley & Sons, Ltd., Publication

Wiley-Blackwell is an imprint of John Wiley & Sons, formed by the merger of Wiley's global Scientific, Technical and Medical business with Blackwell Publishing.

Registered office
John Wiley & Sons Ltd, The Atrium, Southern Gate, Chichester, West Sussex, PO19 8SQ, United Kingdom

Editorial office
John Wiley & Sons Ltd, The Atrium, Southern Gate, Chichester, West Sussex, PO19 8SQ, United Kingdom

For details of our global editorial offices, for customer services and for information about how to apply for permission to reuse the copyright material in this book please see our website at www.wiley.com/wiley-blackwell.

Library of Congress Cataloging-in-Publication Data

Clinical sedation in dentistry / written by N. M. Girdler, C. M. Hill, and K. E. Wilson.
    p.; cm.
  Includes biliographical references and index.
    ISBN 978-1-4051-8069-6 (pbk. : alk. paper)   1. Anesthesia in dentistry.
2. Conscious sedation.   I. Girdler, N. M.   II. Hill, C. M.   III. Wilson, Kathy, 1963–
    [DNLM: 1. Conscious Sedation.   2. Anesthesia, Dental.
WO 460 C641 2009]
  RK510.C55 2009
  617.9′676–dc22
                                                                    2008039839

A catalogue record for this book is available from the British Library.

Set in 10/12pt Utopia by Graphicraft Limited, Hong Kong
Printed in Singapore by Fabulous Printers Pte Ltd

1   2009

Contents

1 Spectrum of anxiety management

▓▓▓▓▓ INTRODUCTION

The aim of this chapter is to introduce the reader to the nature and development of dental anxiety and to provide an understanding of how and why patients behave in the way they do. This forms the basis for the practice of conscious sedation in the management of dental anxiety. The latter part of the chapter explains the development of conscious sedation, the accepted definition and the current guidelines relating to the practice of the technique in dental practice.

One of the main indications for the use of conscious sedation for dental care is 'anxiety'. The prevalence of dental anxiety and phobia is high. The United Kingdom Adult Dental Health Survey of 1998 indicates that 64% of dentate adults identified with being nervous of some kind of dental treatment. The significance of dental anxiety as a barrier towards obtaining dental care, particularly as a result of avoidance, is well recognised. It has also been reported that dental anxiety does not just affect the patient but can have a significant effect on the general dental practitioner who treats the anxious patient. Treating the anxious patient can be a major source of stress for dentists within their daily working environment.

It has been postulated that the aetiology of dental anxiety is multifactorial and modifies and evolves with time. This concept is particularly relevant for the 21st century. With the decline in dental caries in childhood, dental trauma will have a reduced role. Other factors such as the attitudes of family, friends and peers, media influence or the extent to which dental anxiety is part of an overall trait, will become more apparent.

There is a need to understand the individual components of dental anxiety as this will help to increase the dental healthcare worker's awareness in recognising and managing the dentally anxious patient.

FEAR AND ANXIETY AS A NORMAL PHENOMENON

Fear is often considered an essential emotion, augmenting the 'fight or flight' response in times of danger and manifesting as an unpleasant feeling of anxiety or apprehension relating to the presence or anticipation of danger. Fears are found throughout childhood, adolescence and adulthood.

Intense fears in childhood generally subside with maturity and the development of an ability to reason. If they do persist, however, this can result in the development of a 'phobia', a persistent, irrational, intense fear of a specific object, activity or situation. Phobias cause more distress to the patient and are difficult to overcome as they are more resistant to change. Very often some form of psychological/therapeutic intervention is required. Dental phobia invariably leads to dental neglect and total avoidance of dental care and is much more difficult to manage than dental anxiety.

It is therefore important to distinguish between 'phobia' and 'anxiety'.

Anxiety – is a more general non-specific feeling, an unpleasant emotional state, signalling the body to prepare for something unpleasant to happen. Typically anxiety is accompanied by physiological and psychological responses including:

Common physiological responses

- Increased heart rate
- Altered respiration rate
- Sweating
- Trembling
- Weakness/fatigue.

Common psychological responses

- Feelings of impending danger
- Powerlessness
- Tension.

Phobia – may be considered as a form of fear which
- Is irrational and out of proportion to the demands of the situation
- Is beyond voluntary control
- Cannot be explained or reasoned
- Persists over an extended period of time
- Is not age specific.

AETIOLOGY OF DENTAL ANXIETY

The aetiological factors associated with the development of dental anxiety will be dealt with under the following headings:
1. General anxiety and psychological development
2. Gender
3. Traumatic dental experiences
4. Family and peer group influences
5. Defined dental treatment factors.

General anxiety and psychological development

It has been suggested that dental anxiety is a function of personality development associated with feelings of helplessness and abandonment. It is therefore important to consider the age and degree of psychological development of a child when assessing their ability to cope with stressful situations.

As children mature, so their level of understanding increases and the nature of their fears change. In infancy and very early childhood, fear is usually a reaction to the immediate environment, for example loud noises or looming objects. Relating this to the dental environment, it is understandable therefore that a very young child may find the sounds and smells in a dental surgery overwhelming, as well as the sight of the dentist and dental nurse in a white coat.

By the early school years it is suggested that such fears have broadened to include the dark, being alone, imaginary figures, particular people, objects or events (animals and thunder). This could also equate with the dental situation, where a child is perhaps left in the dental chair with the dentist. He or she is unsure of what is going to happen and is unfamiliar with the dental environment.

At about nine years of age, the fear of bodily injury starts to feature strongly. It is clear therefore that for many children the thought of invasive dental procedures may be anxiety-provoking. As the child matures he/she is able to reappraise the potential threat of the situation and may be able to resolve that anxiety.

In adolescence, fear and anxiety are centred on social acceptance and achievement. Some teenagers will be particularly aware of their appearance and possible criticism from peer groups.

In adulthood, although anxieties can develop spontaneously, it is more commonly related to social circumstance or bad experiences.

Gender

There are varying reports and opinions regarding the influence of gender on the aetiology of dental anxiety. Female patients tend to have higher scores for dental anxiety and consider themselves more fearful of dental treatment when compared to men. When considering prevalence studies in children, it would appear that generally girls report more fears than boys. There is much debate as to whether this is due to

- Men being less willing to admit their anxiety
- Women feeling more vulnerable
- Women being more open about their anxieties.

Traumatic dental experience

Negative dental experiences are often quoted as the major factor in the development of dental anxiety with direct negative experiences including painful events, frightening events and embarrassing experiences leading to the development of dental anxiety. Such experiences can occur during childhood, adolescence and adulthood, however, for dental anxiety to develop, it is the nature of the event that appears to be more important than the age at which it occurs.

Traumatic medical experiences can also have a significant relationship with negative dental behaviour and may be important factors in the development of dental anxiety in children.

Family and peer group influences

Influences outside the dentist's control can often heighten dental anxiety. Indiscriminate comments, conversations and negative suggestions about dentistry can induce fear in children and the expectation of an unpleasant experience during dental treatment. Such comments may be made by family members or the child's peers and act as an important source of negative information.

Defined dental treatment factors

Specific dental treatment factors have been defined as the immediate antecedents of dental anxiety, the two most anxiety-arousing being the injection and the drill. Other factors also play a part such as fear of criticism by the dentist, the dentist's attitude and manner and the dental environment. The dentist's attitude may lead to the development of a dentally anxious patient. For example, an abuse of trust by one dentist may result in all dentists being mistrusted. A proposed model for dental fear in children can be seen in Figure 1.1 (Chapman, 1999).

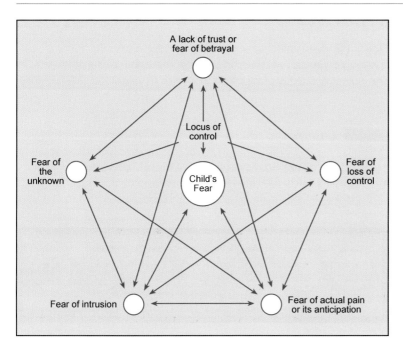

Figure 1.1
A model of dental fear
in children proposed by
Chapman (1999). Taken
from Chapman and
Kirby-Turner (1999).
Reproduced with
Permission from
Wiley-Blackwell.

MEASURING DENTAL ANXIETY

Within dental education the behavioural sciences have
become an increasingly important component. One element
of this has been the application of psychological methods
to study and quantify behaviour and attitudes relevant to
dental care, in particular, dental anxiety and behaviour
during dental treatment. This has included a wide range
of methodological approaches and techniques, including
questionnaires and behaviour measures. Examples of
such measures include children's drawings, observation
of behaviour, visual analogue scales, ratings by dentists
and self-report questionnaires. The most common method
of measuring dental anxiety is by using questionnaires and
rating scales. It is important to ensure the measures used are
reliable, valid and applicable to the population to which they
are aimed.

Commonly used anxiety scales

Adults

- Modified Corah Dental Anxiety Scale
- Visual analogue scale (Figure 1.2)
- Short Dental Anxiety Scale.

Very Anxious ──── X──────────────────────── Not at all Anxious

Figure 1.2 Visual analogue scale – A straight line measuring 10cm, labelled Very Anxious at one end to Not at all Anxious at the other end. The patient is asked to place a X on the line to represent the extent of their anxiety.

Children

- Children's Fear Survey Schedule Dental Subscale
- Smiley Faces Scale (also known as Wong or Venham faces Figure 1.3).

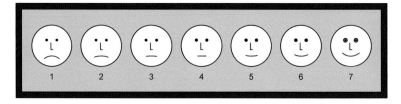

Figure 1.3 Smiley faces anxiety scale – The child is asked to circle the face that best represents how they feel.

SUMMARY

In summary, it is clear that dental anxiety has a multifactorial aetiology comprising age and psychological development, gender of the patient, past traumatic dental and medical experiences, influence of family and peer groups and the immediate antecedents of dental anxiety. All patients will hold their own attitudes and emotions towards the dental situation, as well as their own past dental experiences. The social circumstances and family dynamics will also have an influence on the patient's behaviour and the level of dental anxiety. It is important therefore for those in the dental profession to be aware of this multifactorial aetiology to be able to provide effective behavioural management in the dental setting.

BEHAVIOUR

In order to understand the rationale behind the methods used in treating anxious patients, it is necessary to understand why people behave in the way they do. It is also useful to know how behaviour can be modified in a way that is beneficial for both the patient and the dentist. This can often be achieved without resorting to the use of drugs, allowing long-term solutions to acute problems of behavioural management.

Nature of behaviour

Behaviour may be defined as functioning in a specified, predictable or normal way. In psychological terms, behaviour is a response or series of responses of a person to a given stimulus. The borderline between what is normal (or acceptable) and abnormal (or unacceptable) behaviour is blurred by a host of factors including time, culture, conditioning and other considerations.

The intent of adults would most commonly be to want to behave in a rational and sensible manner, whereas the same intent would not always be present in children and adolescents. It therefore follows that the management of what appears to be similar but abnormal behaviour in the different groups needs to be tackled from a different viewpoint. This illustrates the complexity of the problem when it comes to teaching or learning techniques of behavioural management.

In conclusion, behaviour is a complex issue governed by a multitude of factors, some of which are illustrated in Figure 1.4.

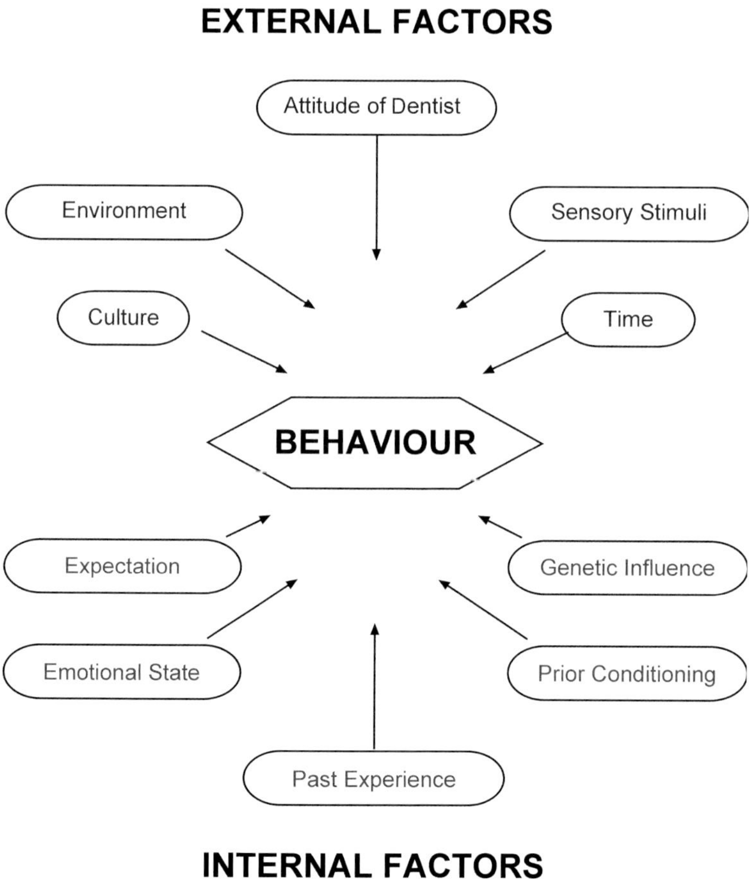

EXTERNAL FACTORS

Attitude of Dentist

Environment

Sensory Stimuli

Culture

Time

BEHAVIOUR

Expectation

Genetic Influence

Emotional State

Prior Conditioning

Past Experience

INTERNAL FACTORS

Figure 1.4
Factors influencing behaviour.

Equally, the management of behaviour is a difficult and extensive subject. However, the successful treatment of any patient depends on a dentist's ability to manage the patient's behaviour satisfactorily and some of the techniques of behavioural management are discussed below.

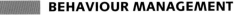 **BEHAVIOUR MANAGEMENT**

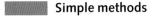 **Simple methods**

There is an element of fear in all unknown situations in the majority of normal individuals. Probably the most important aspect of behavioural management is to ensure that the provoking stimulus is minimised as far as possible. Much of this is common sense and includes paying attention to such factors as room decoration, the way staff are dressed and the playing of gentle music in the background.

Positive distraction: Positive distraction can be applied with the use of ceiling-mounted televisions and personal music systems, as in Figure 1.5.

Although the five sensations of sight, sound, hearing, touch and smell can all be offensive to patients at the dentist, it is undoubtedly the fear of pain which is the most commonly quoted factor that inhibits individuals seeking treatment or which underlies the apparently irrational behaviour of many anxious patients.

Tell, show, do: Simple behavioural management consists of informing verbally and demonstrating practically before

Figure 1.5
Ceiling-mounted television.

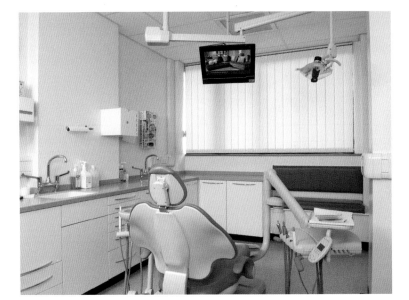

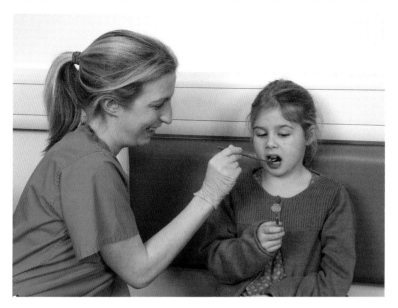

Figure 1.6
By explaining the procedure to the patient and showing them the equipment the patient may feel more confident to proceed with treatment.

actually performing a procedure. This has commonly been interpreted as a 'tell, show, do' sequence and there is good evidence that it is effective for many people (Figure 1.6). It does, however, depend on patients being able to adopt a rational approach to unknown situations. It is unlikely to be very effective in phobic patients or those demonstrating other types of neurotic behaviour.

Permissible deception: Another simple method of behavioural management, and one which is particularly suitable for use in children, is sometimes referred to as 'permissible deception'. An example of this would be the introduction of an infiltration local anaesthetic into an upper premolar region without a patient being told they were having an 'injection'. Providing adequate topical anaesthesia has first been given and the needle is not seen by the patient, abnormal behavioural responses are rarely seen in such situations. In such techniques, it is important not to tell lies but to be 'economical with the truth' using such terms as squirting some numbing water, washing the gums or making the teeth go to sleep.

Successful application of these simple techniques is highly dependent on the confidence of the person applying them. The success of the administration can then be used as a building block on which further steps can be built.

Relaxation techniques: Behavioural response is also heightened by stress, and simple relaxation techniques can be applied to enable tense patients to relax. This may be achieved actively, for example by using progressive relaxation strategies, or passively by using soft background music. It has also been shown that patients perceive the degree of stress being experienced by the dentist and react accordingly, developing heightened responses to any stimuli. It is therefore essential that dentists review their own reactions in difficult or stressful situations and take every action possible to moderate them accordingly.

Systematic desensitisation: This is the most common and potentially most effective psychological technique. It involves gradually acclimatising patients to very minor stimuli and teaching them to relax whilst these are being applied. Once relaxation is achieved the stimulus can be gradually increased usually over a considerable period of time, until even the most feared situation is manageable.

Many dentists intuitively use this approach in treating extremely anxious patients, first of all introducing a mirror and then a probe followed by the use of hand-scalers, tooth-brushing with the dental engine, maxillary infiltration, small restoration, inferior dental block, etc. In many cases it is possible to teach a new set of learned behaviours, replacing the previously maladapted ones.

Hypnosis: The use of hypnosis in dentistry has been slowly increasing as more scientific research and effective postgraduate training have shown potential benefits. A range of techniques can be employed from a simple light hypnotic trance which creates an illusion of relaxation and remoteness, to the use of more complicated phenomena, such as hypno-analgesia, where the effects of a local anaesthetic can be induced through suggestion alone. Hypnosis is a specialised therapeutic technique and should only be practised by those who have received appropriate training.

 SUMMARY

Where behavioural techniques prove unsuccessful, drug therapy may be required to manage patients' anxieties in order for them to be able to comply with dental care. The method of choice for the majority of patients will be conscious sedation. The next section of this chapter will deal with the development of conscious sedation in dentistry, introducing the reader to the history and main principles of its practice.

 SEDATION

In addition to the history and development of conscious sedation, this section also presents the definition and guidelines for sedation in dental practice.

History of sedation

It is difficult to pinpoint the historical beginnings of sedation. The use of alcohol as a narcoleptic is mentioned in the old testament of the Bible and there is evidence that naturally occurring opioids were used over 2,000 years ago in the Eastern world. Modern sedation, however, has evolved over the last hundred years. In the preceding century the practice of anaesthesia itself had been discovered and popularised. This followed the discovery of nitrous oxide by Joseph Priestley in 1772 who himself described the effects produced as 'a highly pleasurable' and 'thrilling' experience.

Some 20 years later Humphrey Davy observed the analgesic properties of nitrous oxide and suggested that it would be suitable for use in surgical procedures. His proposal was largely ignored until Horace Wells, a dental surgeon in Connecticut, USA had a tooth extracted under nitrous oxide. Whether the effect he originally obtained was one of anaesthesia or 'relative analgesia' may never be known for certain. However, since he employed the technique on himself prior to using it on patients, it could be assumed that the effect was one of sedation rather than anaesthesia.

Historically, a number of intravenous drugs have also been used for sedation. Many of the original 'sedation' agents were really general anaesthetic drugs used in smaller doses to try and produce a state of sedation. The drugs included cocktails such as phenobarbitone, pethidine and scopolamine (the Jorgensen technique, named after the Danish/American professor, Niels Jorgensen). Another technique was popularised by the late Stanley Drummond-Jackson and involved giving (allegedly) sub-anaesthetic, multiple doses of the barbiturate methohexitone to induce 'twilight sleep'. Thiopentone, a similar but slightly more potent barbiturate anaesthetic, has also been used in this regard. Needless to say, the border between sedation and anaesthesia was so close that mishaps were inevitable and the practice of intermittent methohexitone was largely discontinued in the early 1970s after one or two fatal episodes. The problem remained that the distinction between sedation and general anaesthesia with all these agents and techniques was extremely narrow and they therefore carried a very fine margin of safety. Accidental anaesthesia with all its attendant dangers was not uncommon.

The fact that sedation practice has largely superseded anaesthetic practice in the UK, was due in no small part to the synthesis of a class of drugs now widely known as the benzodiazepines. The first of these, chlordiazepoxide, was synthesised in 1956 but it was the introduction of diazepam,

Valium®, in both oral and parenteral forms which heralded the arrival of safe sedation. Continued development of sedation drugs and techniques has progressed steadily over the last 50 years. Synthesis of the various benzodiazepines such as midazolam, has been accompanied by extensive research into their mode of action and this is discussed later.

The other area of development has centred on the possibilities of reversible sedation. Modern general anaesthesia relies heavily on such techniques and they have proved extremely effective in regulating anaesthetic depth and duration. The introduction of flumazenil (Anexate®), a reversal agent for the other benzodiazepines, represents a potential first step along this route.

Recent developments in sedation have focused on the possibility of using patient-controlled administration and the use of propofol. This inert phenol derivative is an excellent, short-acting intravenous anaesthetic agent but in theory should suffer from the same objections raised in the administration of intermittent methohexitone. However, the advent of patient-controlled analgesia in post-operative pain control following surgery has raised the possibility that similar mechanisms could be adapted for use in dental surgery. Whether they will ever be appropriate for use by a single operator-sedationist remains to be seen; at the current time such an application cannot be considered permissible due to the development of regulations and guidelines affecting the practice of sedation.

In 1978, the first national report on sedation in the United Kingdom was produced under the chairmanship of Dr W.D. Wylie. It established a definition of conscious sedation which is still the basis of current practice.

The next most significant report concerning sedation was The Poswillo report published in 1990. Through the UK Department of Health, a working party, chaired by Professor Poswillo, was established to review standards for resuscitation, general anaesthesia and conscious sedation in dental practice. The Poswillo report made over 50 recommendations aimed at reducing the risk of adverse health effects or death during dental treatment, including treatment under sedation and general anaesthesia. The recommendations included standards for sedation and general anaesthesia practice; emergency equipment and drugs; training and inspection and registration of premises. Within these guidelines the importance of maintaining communication with the sedated patient is emphasised thereby necessitating a 'conscious sedation' technique. It should be noted that conscious sedation is the only type of sedation applicable to dental practice in the UK.

Current UK practice in conscious sedation

The practice of conscious sedation in dentistry in the UK is regulated by the General Dental Council (GDC) and the Department of Health (DH). Recent guidance applicable to the UK includes *A Conscious Decision* published by the DH in 2000. In 2001 the GDC acted to strengthen the standards relating to conscious sedation in their professional regulations *Maintaining Standards.* More recently two further guidance documents, relating specifically to conscious sedation for dentistry, have been published, one by the Standing Dental Advisory Committee for England and Wales (2003) and one by the National Dental Advisory Committee for Scotland (2006). These documents form the basis for the practice of conscious sedation in the UK, and all members of the dental team should make themselves familiar with the main recommendations.

There is much to be gained from the practice of safe conscious sedation, not just in dentistry but in many other areas of surgery. As with the history of anaesthesia, dentistry has taken the opportunity to lead the way and to point to the ongoing possibilities of further development. This must be based on a sound understanding of the principles and practice of safe sedation, and the remainder of this book aims to give such grounding.

Definition of conscious sedation

The most current guidelines for conscious sedation in United Kingdom define conscious sedation as:

'A technique in which the use of a drug or drugs produces a state of depression of the central nervous system enabling treatment to be carried out, but during which verbal contact with the patient is maintained throughout the period of sedation. The drugs and techniques used to provide conscious sedation for dental treatment should carry a margin of safety wide enough to render loss of consciousness unlikely.'

It should be noted that guidelines on conscious sedation vary at an international level and the reader should be directed to documentation available for his/her own country.

GENERAL ANAESTHESIA

Modern sedation has undoubtedly reduced the number of patients who require a general anaesthetic to tolerate dental treatment, but there remains a significant number who seem unable to tolerate the idea of treatment of any sort unless they are rendered totally unconscious. For this group of people no amount of talking or persuasion will make any difference; unless they are 'knocked out' they will not have any treatment regardless of the degree of pain they are suffering. Whilst this may appear totally irrational, it is no less real and it must be accepted that for those people, a caring professional must provide anaesthetic services at least for the relief of pain and other emergency dental situations. This was the basis of the DH report, *A Conscious Decision*, where guidance was produced for the delivery of safe and effective general anaesthesia for dental treatment. The report also recommended that sedation should be used in preference to general anaesthesia whenever possible.

In the UK, general anaesthesia should now only be provided in hospital-based services where there is access to intensive care facilities. It is banned from general practice in primary care.

SUMMARY

In the first chapter of this book, various methods of patient management have been considered and it is important to remember that many factors will influence decision making, including the patient's age, level of anxiety, relevant medical history, level of co-operation and understanding. It is advisable to adopt a stepped approach when deciding what is in the best interest of the patient, first considering behavioural management techniques and subsequently moving along the scale to sedation or even general anaesthesia in a few cases. Patient management may involve one or more of these modalities depending on the needs of the individual. It is likely that such an approach will be more beneficial in the long term since patients who have general anaesthesia or profound sedation from the outset are less likely to attend recall appointments and have a higher incidence of subsequent dental disease. Those who adopt a progressive approach to sedation, with a view to using it as a treatment modality which can gradually be reduced, are more likely to be successful in their treatment of anxious patients. Sedation should therefore be considered in severely anxious (phobic) patients, moderately anxious patients undergoing difficult or prolonged procedures, anxious child patients, those with certain physical or intellectual disability, and those who may otherwise require a general anaesthetic.

References and further reading

Chapman, H.R. & Kirby-Turner, N.C. (1999) Dental Fear in Children – a proposed model. *British Dental Journal*, **187**(8), 408–412.

Corah, N.L., Gale, E.N., et al. (1978) Assessment of a dental anxiety scale. *Journal of the American Dental Association*, **97**, 816–819.

Department of Health (1990) *General Anaesthesia, Sedation and Resuscitation in Dentistry*. Standing Dental Advisory Committee. Report of an expert Working Party (Chairman: Professor D. Poswillo). London, HMSO.

Department of Health (2000) *A Conscious Decision: A Review of the use of General Anaesthesia and Conscious Sedation in Primary Dental Care*. London, HMSO.

Department of Health (2003) *Conscious Sedation in the Provision of Dental Care*. Standing Dental Advisory Committee. London, HMSO.

Freeman, R.E. (1985) Dental anxiety: a multifactorial aetiology. *British Dental Journal*, **159**, 406.

Freeman, R.E. (1998) A psychodynamic theory for dental phobia. *British Dental Journal*, **184**(4), 170–172.

General Dental Council (2001) *Maintaining Standards*. London, GDC.

Hosey, M.T. & Blinkhorn, A.S. (1995) An evaluation of four methods of assessing the behaviour of anxious child dental patients. *International Journal of Paediatric Dentistry*, **5**, 87–95.

Locker, D., Shapiro, D., et al. (1996) Negative dental experiences and their relationship to dental anxiety. *Community Dental Health*, **13**(2), 86–92.

National Dental Advisory Committee (2006) (*Conscious Sedation in Dentistry*). Dundee, Scottish Dental Clinical Effectiveness Programme.

Newton, T. & Buck, D.J. (2000) Anxiety and pain measures in dentistry. *Journal of the American Dental Association*, **131**, 1449–1457.

Office of National Statistics (1998) *Adult Dental Health Survey: Oral Health in the United Kingdom*. London, HMSO.

Schuurs, A.H.B & Hoogstraten, J. (1993) Appraisal of dental anxiety and fear questionnaires: a review. *Community Dentistry Oral Epidemiology*, **21**, 329–339.

Wilson, K.E. (2006) The use of hypnosis and systematic desensitisation in the management of dental phobia: a case report, *Journal of Disability and Oral Health*, **7**(1), 29–34.

Applied anatomy and physiology

INTRODUCTION

An integrated approach to the anatomy, physiology and, to some extent, the pharmacokinetics of the drugs as they relate to sedation is essential to establish a basis for safe clinical practice. Sound clinical practice must be based on a solid foundation of basic medical science and the following sections address the relevant anatomy, physiology and general pharmacokinetics of sedation. (Pharmacology of the individual agents used for sedation is found in Chapter 4).

All sedatives produce their effects by acting on the brain. The mode of action of a drug is referred to as its pharmacodyanamics, and these are the results of the activity of the drug on the central nervous system. They are essentially the same whether a drug is given orally, intravenously or by inhalation. It is therefore important to have an understanding of applied cardiovascular and respiratory anatomy and physiology relevant to conscious sedation.

CARDIOVASCULAR SYSTEM

The cardiovascular system is a circulatory system comprising the heart, blood vessels and the cells and plasma that make up the blood. The blood vessels of the body represent a closed delivery system, which transports blood around the body, circulating substances such as oxygen, nutrients and hormones to the organs and tissues. The circulatory system also acts to remove metabolic wastes such as carbon dioxide and other unwanted products. The heart is a specialised muscle, the principal function of which is to act as a pump to maintain the circulation of blood within the blood vessels. The three main types of blood vessel are:

Arteries: The afferent blood vessels carrying blood away from the heart. The walls (outer structure) of arteries contain smooth muscle fibres that contract and relax in response to the sympathetic nervous system.

Veins: The efferent blood vessels returning blood to the heart. The walls (outer structure) of veins consist of three layers of tissues that are thinner and less elastic than the corresponding layers of arteries. Veins include valves that aid the return of blood to the heart by preventing blood from flowing in the reverse direction.

The basic structure of the vessel wall (see Figure 2.1) is similar in all blood vessels with the *tunica intima* or endothelium lining the vessel's lumen. Externally is a connective tissue, the *tunica adventitia* which is slightly thicker in arteries. The middle layer is a layer of smooth muscle, the *tunica media*, which is much thicker in arteries and which is largely responsible for the peripheral control of blood pressure. The endothelial lining of veins is enveloped to form valves which, with external muscle influence, assist in propelling blood back to the heart (valves are rarely taken into consideration during venepuncture, but they can be used to benefit or to hinder successful cannulation of a vein).

Capillaries: These are narrow, thin-walled blood vessels (approximately 5–20 micrometres in diameter) that connect arteries to veins. Capillary networks exist in most of the tissues and organs of the body, and the narrow cell walls allow exchange of material between the contents of the capillary and the surrounding tissue. The networks are the site of gas, nutrient and waste exchange between the blood and the respiring tissues.

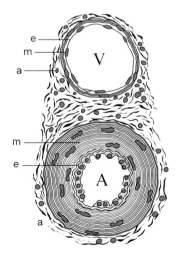

Figure 2.1

Transverse section of an artery and vein. **A**, Artery, lined with nucleated endothelium **(e)**. Underneath the endothelium is the elastic lamina muscle layer **(m)**. The muscle layer is surrounded by connective tissue fibres, the adventitia **(a)**. **V**, Vein, has thin endothelial lining **(e)**, under which is a very thin muscle layer **(m)**. The adventia **(a)** is similar to the artery.

The heart

The heart is composed of cardiac muscle; involuntary muscle tissue only is found within this organ. It is a small but complex organ. The left side of the heart delivers oxygenated blood, via the aorta, to the systemmic circulation. The right side of the heart receives deoxygenated blood (Figure 2.2).

Figure 2.2
Cross-section of the heart illustrating the flow of blood through the chambers and large vessels.

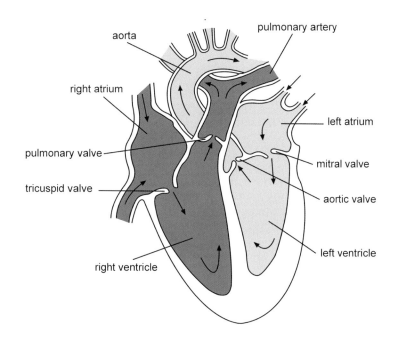

aorta

pulmonary artery

right atrium

left atrium

pulmonary valve

mitral valve

tricuspid valve

aortic valve

left ventricle

right ventricle

Cardiac cycle

The cardiac cycle is defined as the sequence of pressure and volume changes that take place during cardiac activity. The time of a cycle in a healthy adult is approximately 0.9 seconds, although it varies considerably, giving an average pulse rate of around 70 beats per minute (bpm). There are two elements of the cardiac cycle:
- Systole: rapid contraction of heart, 0.3 sec
- Diastole: resting phase, 0.5 sec.

Heart rate (HR): The number of ventricular contractions occurring in one minute.
Stroke volume (SV): The volume of blood ejected in one ventricular contraction, approximately 70ml.
Cardiac output (CO): The amount of blood ejected from one ventricle during one minute (i.e. stroke volume × heart rate). The cardiac output of the right ventricle passes through the

lungs, whilst the output from the left ventricle passes into the aorta and is distributed to the organs and tissues.

The cardiac output is a product of stroke volume and heart rate described by the following equation: $CO = SV \times HR$ and is directly affected by three factors:

- Filling pressure of the right side of the heart
- Resistance to outflow (peripheral resistance)
- Functional state of the heart-lung unit.

Conduction system

The aim of the conduction system is to enable atrial and ventricular contraction to be coordinated efficiently. Contraction or depolarisation of the heart is initiated via impulses generated in the sinoatrial node (SAN) and conducted through adjacent atrial muscle cells, causing systole in both atria. The depolarisation continues on to the atrioventicular node (AVN). These two nodes have their own inherent rhythm of: SAN 80 bpm and AVN 40 bpm. The AVN conducts the impulse on via the Bundle of His to the ventricles. These nerves divide into Purkinje fibres throughout the ventricles, and the result is to depolarise the whole ventricle (Figure 2.3).

The SAN is considered to be the heart's pacemaker and is under the influence of the sympathetic and parasympathetic nervous systems. The parasympathetic system (via the Vagus nerve) acts to slow the heart whilst the sympathetic system increases the heart rate and volume intensity.

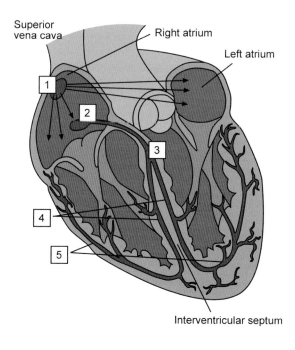

Interventricular septum

Figure 2.3
Conduction system of the heart: **1**- Sinoatrial node; **2**- Atrioventricular node; **3**- Bundle of His; **4**- Bundle branches; **5**- Purkinje fibres.

As well as the nervous and chemical stimulation, there are hormonal influences on the cardiovascular system. The kidneys produce renin which converts to angiotensin II which is an extremely powerful vasoconstrictor. In addition, the adrenal medulla can produce central release of catecholamines which simulate the action of the β receptors and induce sympathetic stimulation of the heart. Finally, there is a hormone released by the vessel endothelium known as endothelium-derived relaxing factor (EDRF) which causes vasodilatation.

Thus, control of the cardiovascular system can be seen to consist of a highly complex series of mechanisms that can easily be disturbed by external factors such as sedation. In young and healthy individuals the compensatory mechanisms are more than adequate to deal with this, but in the frail and elderly cardiovascular problems develop much more readily and allowance should always be made for this. This may also be true for those recovering from serious illnesses or who may be debilitated for any other reason.

Heart rate

The heart rate will vary depending on age, anxiety and the presence of systemic pathology. Average heart rates are illustrated in Table 2.1.

Tachycardia refers to a rapid heart rate (>100 bpm in adults). Tachycardia may be a perfectly normal physiological response to stress or exercise. However, depending on the mechanism of the tachycardia and the health status of the patient, tachycardia may be harmful and require medical treatment.

Tachycardia can be harmful in two ways. First, when the heart beats too rapidly, it may pump blood less efficiently. Second, the faster the heart beats, the more oxygen and nutrients it requires. As a result, the patient may feel out of breath or, in severe cases, suffer chest pain. This can be especially problematic for patients with ischaemic heart disease.

Table 2.1	Average heart rates		
Age	Av. HR	Lower limit	Site
Infant <1yr	120	60	brachial
Child <8yr	100	50	carotid
Adult	72	40/50	carotid

Bradycardia is defined as a resting heart rate <60 bpm in adults. It is rarely symptomatic until the rate drops below 50 bpm. It is quite common for trained athletes to have slow resting heart rates, and this should not be considered abnormal if the individual has no associated symptoms.

Bradycardia can result from a number of causes which can be classified as cardiac or non-cardiac. Non-cardiac causes are usually secondary, and can involve drug use or misuse; metabolic or endocrine issues (especially related to the thyroid), neurologic factors, and situational factors such as prolonged bed rest. Cardiac causes include acute or chronic ischaemic heart disease, vascular heart disease or valvular heart disease.

The blood is driven through the vascular system by the pressure produced on ejection of the blood from the ventricles followed by the elastic response of the major arteries (Figure 2.4).

Blood pressure

Blood pressure refers to the force exerted by circulating blood on the walls of blood vessels. It is a function of cardiac output and peripheral vascular resistance. Blood pressure is important

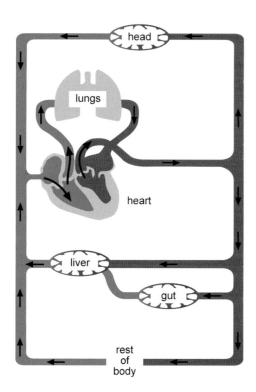

Figure 2.4
Circulation of blood through the vascular system.

as it maintains blood flow to and from the heart, the brain, kidneys and other major organs and tissues.

The systolic pressure is defined as the peak pressure in the arteries, which occurs near the beginning of the cardiac cycle. The diastolic pressure is the lowest pressure (at the resting phase of the cardiac cycle).

Typical values for a resting, healthy adult human are approximately 100–130mmHg systolic and 60–85mmHg diastolic (average 120/80mmHg). These measures of blood pressure are not static but undergo natural variations from one heartbeat to another and throughout the day. They also change in response to stress, nutritional factors, drugs or disease. Hypertension refers to blood pressure being abnormally high; hypotension, when it is abnormally low.

Control of blood pressure

Blood pressure (BP) is affected by the peripheral vascular resistance (PR) and the cardiac output (CO). Peripheral resistance results from the natural elasticity of the arteries and is an essential feature of the circulatory system. When the heart contracts, blood enters the arteries faster than it can leave, resulting in the arteries stretching from the pressure. As the reverse pressure begins to exceed the ejectory pressure, the aortic valve closes and the atria refill.

The factors affecting blood pressure are many and include:
- Baroreceptor mechanism
- Carbon dioxide
- Hypoxia and chemoreceptors
- Respiratory centre
- Sensory nerves
- Higher centres
- Drugs.

Each of these will be briefly considered.
- *Baroreceptor mechanism*: Baroreceptors are pressure receptors found in the aortic arch and carotid sinus. Increased baroreceptor activity inhibits vasomotor centre (VMC) activity in the brain, leading to arterial vasodilatation, a lowering in PR and a consequent fall in BP. Similarly, decreased baroreceptor activity disinhibits VMC activity leading to arterial vasoconstriction, a rise in PR, with a corresponding rise in BP. Receptors can also be stimulated artificially, for example external pressure on the neck by high shirt collars.
- *Carbon dioxide*: Carbon dioxide (CO_2) is essential for the functioning of the VMC. A decrease in CO_2 leads to

decreased VMC activity and a fall in BP, with an increase in CO_2 having the opposite effect.

- *Sensory nerves*: Pain modifies the activity of the VMC, with mild pain increasing VMC activity, leading to an increase in BP. Severe pain decreases VMC activity and may lead to a drop in BP. In this situation the body is acting in a protective way. The mechanisms by which this occurs are complex.
- *Higher centres*: Emotional stress or excitement often increases BP by affecting the VMC and also increases cardiac output. In emotional shock there may be a fall in BP, e.g. at the sight of blood.
- *Drugs*: The majority of anaesthetic and sedative drugs cause a drop in BP by reducing the brain's ability to respond to stimuli to change BP, and the muscle relaxant effect therefore leads to a reduction in PR. It is therefore essential to monitor blood pressure throughout procedures involving general anaesthesia or sedation.

Irregularities in blood pressure

1. Hypertension (high blood pressure) – Hypertension exists when the the blood pressure is chronically elevated. It is usually defined as a resting blood pressure above 140/90mmHG in a patient aged less than 50 years or above 160/95mmHG in older patients. Predisposing factors include:
- Age (blood pressure rises with age)
- Obesity
- Excessive alcohol intake
- Genetic susceptibility.

2. Hypotension (low blood pressure) – Hypotension results if the systolic blood pressure falls below 80mmHg. It often presents with the features of shock, including tachycardia and cold and clammy skin. The common symptoms of hypotension are lightheadedness and dizziness and, if the blood pressure is sufficiently low, syncope (fainting) often occurs. This situation is not uncommon in the dental surgery and is normally easily managed.

Low blood pressure in patients presenting at assessment may be due to autonomic failure as a result of drugs that interfere with autonomic function, e.g. tricyclic antidepressants, or drugs that interfere with peripheral vasoconstriction including nitrates and calcium antagonists.

Importance of blood pressure in the dental patient

Dental treatment is perceived as a stressful situation by many patients and in this situation blood pressure may be elevated.

This becomes an issue mainly in patients with underlying cardiovascular disease and can predispose to cardiovascular events such as myocardial infarction, strokes, etc.

▨▨▨▨ VASCULAR ANATOMY OF UPPER LIMB RELEVANT TO SEDATION

An understanding of the anatomy of the arm is important since the most commonly used veins for cannulation are the superficial veins of the dorsum of the hand (Figure 2.5), and the anticubital fossa (Figure 2.6).

It is important to note that in the antecubital fossa (Figure 2.6) there are three important structures that must be avoided:

Figure 2.5
Veins of the dorsum of the hand.

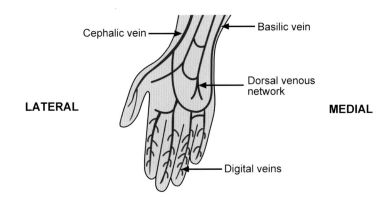

Figure 2.6
Antecubital fossa illustrating the three important structures to be aware of: brachial artery, median nerve and bicipital aponeurosis.

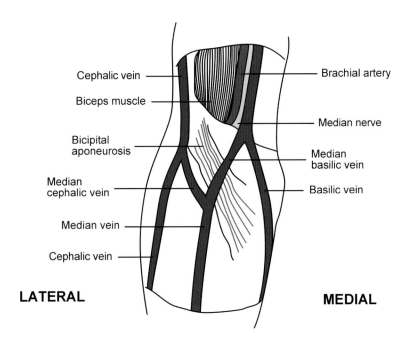

- The brachial artery
- The median nerve
- Bicipital aponeurosis.

Fortunately, all three are to be found on the medial aspect of the fossa and so injections lateral to the easily palpable biceps tendon in order to avoid these structures.

RESPIRATORY SYSTEM

The respiratory system facilitates oxygenation of the blood with a concomitant removal from the circulation of carbon dioxide and other gaseous metabolic waste. Anatomically, the respiratory system consists of the nose, pharynx, larynx, trachea, bronchi and bronchioles. The bronchioles lead to the respiratory zone of the lungs which consists of respiratory bronchioles, alveolar ducts and the alveoli, the multi-lobulated sacs in which most of the gas exchange occurs.

Upper airway

The upper airway consists of the nose and pharynx. The pharynx is divided into three sections: nasopharynx, oropharynx and laryngopharynx (Figure 2.7).

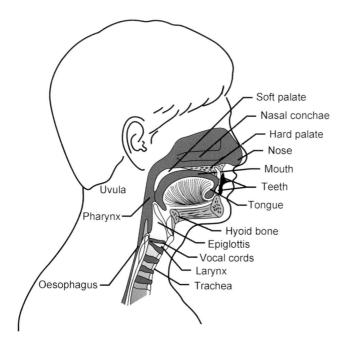

Figure 2.7
Upper airway.

Figure 2.8
Lower airway.

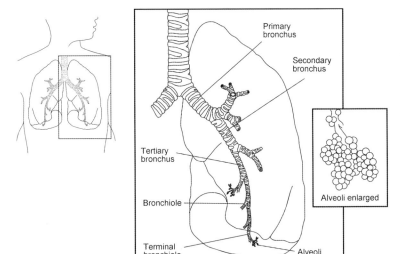

Lower airway

The lower airway (Figure 2.8) consists of the:
Larynx – The mucosa of the larynx (voice box) is very sensitive, and if irritated the cough reflex is initiated by the strong muscles surrounding the structure. This acts as a protective mechanism preventing the entry of foreign objects.
Trachea – The trachea is a continuation of the larynx beginning at the level of the sixth cervical vertebra. It is approximately 11cm long with a diameter of 20mm. The trachea bifurcates into the right and left bronchi.
Bronchi – The left bronchus emerges at an angle of approximately 45 degrees from the trachea. The right bronchus branches off at an angle of 25 degrees; it is approximately 2.5cm in length and, for this reason, inhaled foreign bodies tend to be directed to the right lung. The main bronchi then divide into smaller branches to supply the lobes of the lungs.
Bronchioles – The bronchioles are a continued division of the bronchi which themselves divide further into the alveolar ducts, alveolar sacs and alveoli. It is within the capillary beds of the alveoli that exchange between air and carbon dioxide in the blood occurs.

Respiration

The process of respiration consists of external and internal mechanisms.

- *External respiration* – where there is an exchange of gases between lungs and blood
- *Internal respiration* – involving exchange of gases between blood and cells.

With an inhalation sedation agent, the gas must enter the lungs, cross the alveolar membranes to be absorbed into the blood, be pumped round the left side of the heart into the arterial blood before reaching the tissues of the body. There are, therefore, three aspects of this process: entry into the lungs; circulation to the tissues; and excretion or removal from the body.

Control of respiration

Ventilation of the lungs is carried out by the muscles of respiration and is under the control of the autonomic nervous system from part of the brain stem, the medulla oblongata and the pons. This area of the brain forms the respiration regulatory centre (Figure 2.9).

   This control centre receives information from a variety of sources including other brain receptors, the lungs, the blood vessels and the respiratory muscles. In addition, the respiratory centre receives information from various chemoreceptors in the medulla which monitor the pH of the cerebrospinal fluid.

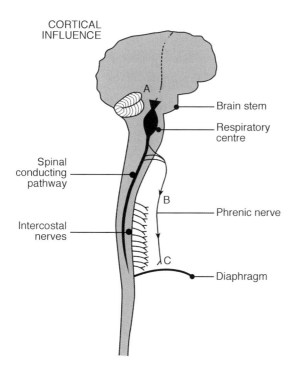

CORTICAL INFLUENCE

Brain stem

Respiratory centre

Spinal conducting pathway

Phrenic nerve

Intercostal nerves

Diaphragm

Figure 2.9
The control of respiration is influenced at several points. At point A, the respiratory centre is affected by all modern sedatives. At points B and C, the phrenic nerve and neuromuscular junction respectively, the influences are less profound.

Changes in pH are largely influenced by the rise and fall of
carbon dioxide levels since increased carbon dioxide (CO_2)
availability leads to an increase in hydrogen ion availability
(and a lowering of pH) as carbonic acid forms.

$$CO_2 + H_2O = H_2CO_3 = H^+ + HCO_3^-$$

In healthy individuals, the respiratory centre is thus able to
provide very rapid responses to changes in pH or, in effect,
partial pressure of carbon dioxide ($PaCO_2$) which it represents.
Indeed, a rise of only 1mm Hg in the $PaCO_2$ will result in an
increase in the ventilation rate of about 2.5 litres/minute.
However, long-term exposure of the chemoreceptors to
chronically high $PaCO_2$ levels results in a diminished response
and would be seen, for instance, in patients suffering from
chronic bronchitis. There are, in addition, chemoreceptors
of a different type within the carotid bodies and these are
generously supplied with arterial blood. They respond to
falls in oxygen saturation (PaO_2) but their effect on the
respiration rate is far less dramatic than that of the CO_2
receptors, since they require a more substantial reduction
of the PaO_2 before they have a clinically significant effect on
the respiration rate.

Information for the respiratory centre is also derived from
stretch receptors in the lungs and respiratory muscles. All this
information is used to process the control of breathing depth
for regular breathing. Complex mechanisms (e.g. sneezing,
coughing) are initiated by different receptors in the respiratory
tract mucosa.

Finally, there is some control of breathing in the higher
centres and indeed, control of breathing can be made a
voluntary action – a feature which is used in some relaxation
techniques. Normally, however, breathing and the processes of
respiration occur involuntarily and, if fear or emotion threaten
to make them too irregular, some attempt at voluntary control
can be made.

Having processed the information from the chemoreceptors
in the medulla, those in the carotid bodies and the information
from the tactile receptors in the diaphragm, the process of
breathing is initiated along the phrenic nerve. In normal
breathing this involves contraction and relaxation of the
diaphragm. Combined with the contraction of the intercostal
muscles, the rib cage is pulled upwards and outwards. This
increases the internal volume of the thorax and creates a
sub-atmospheric pressure which draws air in through the
nose and/or mouth, past the pharynx, larynx and trachea to
the bronchi. The bronchi comprise multiple bronchioles
and alveoli (clusters of capillary-lined tissue which allow the

perfusion of gases). The whole of this section of the respiratory process is termed inspiration.

Inspiration

Inhalation is initiated by the diaphragm and supported by the external intercostal muscles. When the diaphragm contracts, the rib cage expands and the contents of the abdomen are moved downward. This results in a larger thoracic volume, which in turn causes a decrease in intrathoracic pressure. As the pressure in the chest falls, air moves into the conducting zone. Here, the air is filtered, warmed, and humidified as it flows to the lungs.

Expiration

Expiration is generally a passive process where, the diaphragm and intercostal muscles relax and the rib cage returns passively to its original shape. The lungs have a natural elasticity; as they recoil from the stretch of inhalation, air flows back out until the pressures in the chest and the atmosphere reach equilibrium.

The alveolar blood, previously rich in carbon dioxide, has continued circulating and diffusing CO_2 out of the blood; the loss of oxygen from the inspired air results in a gas mixture containing 5% carbon dioxide and only 16% oxygen; the nitrogen content remains virtually constant.

The processes of inspiration and expiration comprise the process of external respiration. Inspiration is a highly muscular process whilst expiration is relatively passive, thus explaining why people with asthma (bronchial spasm) find breathing out much harder than breathing in when they are suffering an attack.

If there is obstruction of the upper airway, this may result in 'paradoxical respiration'. Paradoxical or 'see-saw' respiration is the result of the diaphragm and intercostal muscles contracting in an attempt to increase the size of the thorax. When this does not occur (due to the obstruction) the dimensions actually decrease whilst the abdominal volume increases. This is the exact reverse of what would be anticipated during the inspiratory phase and the exact opposite occurs in the expiratory phase, hence the terminology.

Lung volumes

A healthy adult will inspire and expire about 450ml of air each breath, a figure known as the tidal volume. In the course of a minute, about 12 breaths would be taken, known as the respiration rate. This allows the calculation of the minute volume which can be expressed as:

MINUTE VOLUME = TIDAL VOLUME × RESPIRATION RATE

A simple calculation (450ml × 12) shows this to be just over 5 litres per minute in a healthy adult, although allowances need to be made for size and other factors. Of that volume only two-thirds ever reaches the alveoli of the lungs where it is available for gas transfer. The remaining part, occupying the nose, pharynx, trachea and bronchi, which is not available for gas transfer, is known as the dead space and is normally 150ml. The dead space increases with chronic lung disease, e.g. bronchitis, asthma. The relative volumes can be seen in Table 2.2 and are illustrated graphically in Figure 2.10.

Lung entry

The effect of a gas (i.e. its degree of activity or depth of sedation) depends on several factors but the speed of onset is principally dependent on its partial pressure at the site of

Table 2.2	Lung volumes
Characteristic	Volume
Tidal volume – normal breath	450 – 500 ml
Vital capacity – maximum inspiration to expiration	3.0 to 5.0 litres
Residual volume – amount left after forced expiration	1.5 litres
Total lung capacity – The sum of the vital capacity and the residual volume	
Inspiratory reserve volume – air which an individual can force into the lungs during breathing (approximately)	3 litres
Expiratory reserve volume – The amount of air that can be forced out of the lungs by an individual after a normal breath	1.5 litres
Functional residual capacity – The amount of air which remains after quiet expiration (approximately)	3 litres

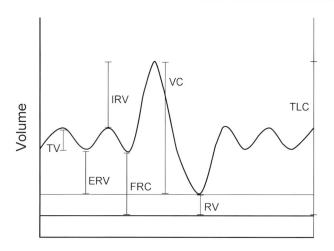

Figure 2.10
Graphical representation
of lung volumes:
TV – Tidal volume;
ERV – Expiratory reserve
volume; **IRV** – Inspiratory
reserve volume;
FRC – Functional reserve
capacity; **VC** – Vital
capacity; **RV** – Residual
volume; **TLC** – Total lung
capacity.

action. Partial pressure may be thought of as the force with which a gas is trying to come out of a solution in which it has been dissolved. In general terms it is inversely proportional to the solubility of a gas. Thus, nitrous oxide which has a very low solubility results in a rapid rise in partial pressure. The halogenated vapours (e.g. ethrane, isoflurane) have much higher solubilities and therefore respond with much slower rises in partial pressure.

The importance of understanding this concept cannot be emphasised enough since it is relevant to both the potency of the gas or vapour and its speed of action. The less soluble gases or vapours are normally less potent but quicker acting. For this reason, a relatively insoluble gas like nitrous oxide is ideal for use in sedation since it combines two of the ideal properties for an inhalation agent, i.e. it is quick acting but not excessively potent. By virtue of its mode of action, it is dependent on the process of respiration for initial entry into the lungs and some understanding of the process of respiration is essential.

Circulation to the tissues

As mentioned earlier, an inhalation agent must enter the lungs and cross the alveolar membranes to be absorbed into the blood (the processes relating to intravenous agents will be considered in the next section). During the induction of sedation each breath of nitrous oxide results in a small but incremental rise in the partial pressure. Partial pressure is dependent on the solubility (or lack thereof) of the gas and this is expressed as the blood-gas coefficient. Blood-gas or (partition coefficient) is defined as the ratio of the number of molecules of a gas in the blood phase to the number of molecules in the gaseous phase at a point of equilibrium. Soluble agents have higher values (e.g. ether is about 13) whilst gases of low solubility have low values (e.g. nitrous oxide is 0.47).

As the nitrous oxide dissolves in the alveolar blood it is rapidly transported away via the pulmonary vein to the left side of the heart. It is then ejected into the circulation through the aorta and thence via the arteries and arterioles to the capillary blood vessels where gas exchange with the tissues takes place. The speed of this process is dependent on the cardiac output, the volume of blood ejected into the circulation each minute from the left ventricle. If the cardiac output is high, a relatively large volume of blood also flows though the lungs. This means that the same amount of gas (i.e. each tidal volume) is taken into this larger volume resulting a lower concentration (concentration = mass per unit volume). Conversely, patients with a lower cardiac output have less blood available for gas diffusion and therefore respond with a more rapid rise in partial pressure. This helps to explain why nitrous oxide is most effective when used to reinforce suggestion and when prior relaxation has helped to reduce heart rate and thus cardiac output. This also has a direct effect in reducing the patient's blood pressure since this is a factor of cardiac output and peripheral vascular resistance. There is some debate about what constitutes a 'safe' blood pressure but the greatest danger in this regard tends to be with sudden and unexpected changes, rather than the actual values.

Oxygen and carbon dioxide exchange

Whilst the processes of inspiration and expiration comprise external respiration (the means by which oxygen and carbon dioxide are interchanged in the lungs) it is the process of internal respiration (the means by which oxygen and carbon dioxide are interchanged in the tissues) which is perhaps most significant. In this respect, oxygen is of fundamental importance since the production of adenosine triphosphate (ATP) runs much more efficiently and for much longer when supplied with oxygen (aerobic metabolism) than when oxygen is not available or in short supply (anaerobic respiration).

An understanding of the passage of oxygen into and out of the bloodstream can be derived from consideration of partial pressures. Atmospheric pressure is usually between 750–770mmHg or approximately 100 kilopascals (kPa) (752mmHg = 100kPa). Oxygen comprises nearly 21% of the atmospheric volume and so has a partial pressure of 21kPa as it enters the nose. In the lungs the presence of water vapour lowers the partial pressure of the oxygen by about 5% to just

under 20kPa. Since blood will saturate with an oxygen partial
pressure of 16kPa (120mmHg), this is more than adequate to
create a sufficient gradient across which the oxygen can diffuse
into the blood, principally (but not entirely) the haemoglobin
of the red blood cells. The gradient must exist, however, since
the oxygen does not get 'sucked' into the blood. The circulating
venous blood has a residual oxygen content represented by a
partial pressure of about 5–6kPa (40mmHg). After saturation,
this level (i.e. the arterial PaO_2) increases to 13kPa in a process
known as arterialisation. Within the tissues the oxygen
saturation varies, with some organs being oxygen rich (e.g.
liver, muscles at rest) and some relatively low (e.g. fat). Oxygen
leaves the blood when the pressure gradient is negative and
enters the blood when it is positive.

The relationship between PaO_2 and haemoglobin saturation
is well known as a dissociation curve and can be influenced by a
variety of factors (Figure 2.11).

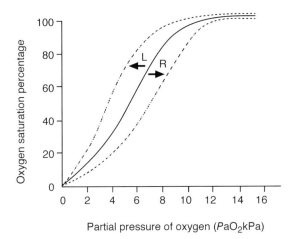

Partial pressure of oxygen (PaO_2kPa)

Figure 2.11
Oxygen/haemoglobin
dissociation curve. The
curve can be displaced
to the left or the right by
systemic influences.

Shifts to the left result in lower availability of oxygen to the
tissues; shifts to the right increase the availability. An
understanding of the significance of the S-shaped dissociation
curve is also important since, like a car rolling down an incline,
the pace of acceleration increases rapidly as the gradient rises.

In the healthy adult every gram of haemoglobin is capable of
absorbing nearly 1.4ml of oxygen. Some simple maths enables
the total volume of oxygen in the blood to be calculated but a
small allowance must also be made for the oxygen dissolved in
plasma (about 3ml per litre). The concept of oxygen availability
is important in all aspects of sedation, both inhalation and
intravenous, and is summarised in Figure 2.12.

OXYGEN AVAILABILITY = ARTERIAL OXYGEN CONTENT x CARDIAC OUTPUT

ARTERIAL OXYGEN CONTENT = PLASMA OXYGEN + HAEMOGLOBIN OXYGEN

PLASMA OXYGEN CONTENT = 3ml/l AT 37° AND 13kPa

HAEMOGLOBIN OXYGEN CONTENT = HAEMOGLOBIN CONCENTRATION x 1.39 x % SATURATION

Figure 2.12
Principles involved in
oxygen availability.

INTRAVENOUS DRUGS AND EXCRETION

The vast majority of intravenous drugs are, after injection into the blood stream, carried in the blood plasma. Very few drugs bind to the blood cells in the way that, for example, oxygen does. The plasma level (or concentration) causes a diffusion gradient between the circulation and the tissues, resulting in the drug crossing the tissue (or lipid) membranes to the site of action in the brain (it should be noted, of course, that the drugs cross other lipid membranes and not solely those in the brain).

When a drug is injected it is present in the plasma in its manufactured form, i.e. dissolved in water or some other solvent. The drug may be ionised or un-ionised but drugs cannot penetrate lipid membranes in an ionised state. Only un-ionised drugs are lipid soluble and only lipid-soluble drugs can penetrate lipid membranes. A drug may also be bound to a plasma protein when it also becomes ineffective at the site of action. An injected drug may therefore be:

• free but ionised
• bound to plasma proteins
• free and un-ionised.

Only the last category will be effective. However, there is free interchange between the various states and this can have a dramatic effect on the mode and duration of action of a drug (Figure 2.13).

Figure 2.13
The distribution of an
intravenously injected
drug.

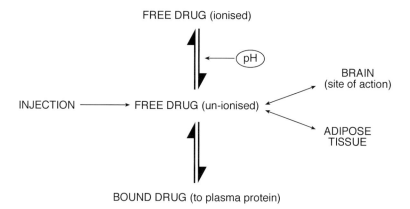

Redistribution

Once circulating in the blood, a process of balancing the diffusion gradients occurs and this is generally referred to as redistribution – the passage of un-ionised lipid soluble unbound drug into body tissues, mainly fat. This process largely explains the principle of the 'alpha half-life' – $T1/2\alpha$ – the time taken for the serum concentration to fall by 50%. The $T1/2\alpha$ is a useful clinical concept since it refers to the observed effects in a patient. Once a drug has been redistributed to the extent that its serum concentration has fallen below a therapeutic level, the effect of the drug appears to have worn off.

Elimination

Following metabolism of the drug it is excreted from the body. The time taken to remove half the drug from the body is referred to as the beta half-life – $T1/2\beta$. The more quickly a drug is metabolised, the more the $T1/2\alpha$ and $T1/2\beta$ converge.

Onset of action

The onset of action of an intravenous drug is dependent on four factors, two of which are the same as for the inhalation agents. These are:
1. ***The total dose injected***: greater plasma levels obviously being achieved with higher doses
2. ***The duration of injection***: a shorter the injection time resulting in a more rapid rise in plasma level
3. ***The cardiac output***: see earlier
4. ***The circulating blood volume***: smaller blood volumes result in higher concentrations.

Recovery

Recovery is also affected by the last two factors but principally by:
1. ***Redistribution***: The rate and extent of redistribution of the drug within the tissues
2. ***Metabolism***: The rate and extent of liver metabolism
3. ***Excretion***: The rate and extent of excretion.

Most intravenous agents are highly lipid soluble and, despite the less than generous blood supply to the adipose tissue compared with the brain or liver, the sheer mass of fat causes an increased amount of the drug to be taken into the adipose tissues. This subsequently causes a reversal of the blood to brain diffusion gradient, moving the drug back from the brain into the blood. Once the plasma concentration drops below the therapeutic level the patient begins to recover.

It cannot be stressed enough, however, that this does not represent a point at which the drug has left the body; a fact which may have dire consequences if further increments of a drug are added without allowing for the already circulating drug doses. This has two potential effects. First, the dose of any increment required is likely to be considerably less than would be expected, and second, because of the reduced pressure gradients already present between the plasma and the tissues, recovery would be more prolonged than anticipated.

Recovery from a drug is therefore dependent on two physiological processes (Figure 2.14). Redistribution of the drug may allow clinical recovery from a drug's effects but metabolism (and excretion) is essential to remove the drug from the body's tissues.

These two factors partly determine the profile of a drug's action – its pharmacokinetics – whilst the actual mechanisms by which a drug actually works – what it does – are its pharmacodyanamics. The details of these processes vary considerably with different drugs and largely determine the properties of an agent.

Drugs which circulate in the plasma are at some stage removed from the body. Intravenous drugs are most commonly metabolised in the liver producing breakdown products known as metabolites. Some of these are themselves active drugs and, unless they are passed into the bile and not reabsorbed, they may produce secondary effects (as will be seen later, this is a well known feature of some of the benzodiazepines). Normally the metabolites produced by the liver are delivered back into the plasma where they again pass via several diffusion gradients to the kidneys for excretion. It is only when a drug

Figure 2.14
Recovery from intravenous sedation occurs initially by redistribution of the drug into adipose tissue followed by elimination of the drug by the liver and kidney.

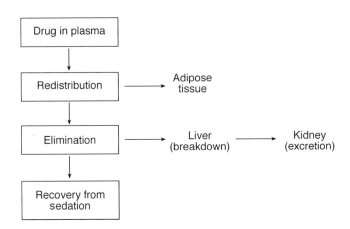

and all its metabolites have been completely cleared from the body that total recovery can be said to be complete. In some cases this may take days or occasionally even weeks to occur, despite an agent appearing to be effective clinically for perhaps only a few hours. Thus, the importance of understanding the relationship between the anatomical and physiological function and the pharmacokinetics of a drug can be seen to be more important than just theoretical academia.

References and further reading

Ellis, H., Feldman, J. & Harrop-Griffiths, W. (2004) *Anatomy for Anaesthetists.* Oxford, Blackwell Scientific Publications.

Pinsky, M.R. (1997) *Applied Cardiovascular Physiology.* New York, Springer.

Snell, R.S. (1995) *Clinical Anatomy for Medical Students,* 5th edn. Boston, Little, Brown.

Stoelting, R.K. & Hillier, S.C. (eds) (2006) *Pharmacology and Physiology in Anesthetic Practice.* 4th edn. Philadelphia, Lippincott Williams & Wilkins.

3 Patient assessment

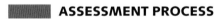 **INTRODUCTION**

Careful pre-sedation appraisal will optimise the safety and effectiveness of sedation. Patient selection and assessment is an essential prerequisite to the success of subsequent treatment under conscious sedation. The assessment provides an opportunity to obtain relevant information from the patient to determine suitability for both sedation and dental treatment. It allows the patient to discuss their treatment with the clinician and for both to establish a mutual rapport. This is of particular importance for severely anxious patients who may have lost confidence with the dental environment through previous negative experiences. Such patients need to be managed with care and reassurance to regain their trust and co-operation.

This chapter will consider all aspects of the assessment process and discuss the relevance of certain medical conditions in the delivery of conscious sedation.

ASSESSMENT PROCESS

Setting

A specific appointment should be arranged, whenever possible, for the pre-operative assessment separate to the treatment day. Ideally this visit should take place in a non-clinical, and therefore non-threatening, environment. It is important to create a calm and relaxed atmosphere to help reassure patients and put them at ease.

History taking

The accepted sequence of history taking, followed by examination is no different from the assessment of any patient, but there should be special emphasis on the need for sedation, reasons for treatment under sedation and the patient's fitness to receive sedation. Only when all of this information is available can an individual treatment plan be formulated. It is also important to gain indirect information about patients from the way they respond to questioning and, even more importantly, from the initial examination.

The history must include details of the nature of the patient's dental anxiety, particular difficulty with dental treatment, e.g. a gag reflex, the past dental history and current dental symptoms, a thorough medical history and information on social circumstances. The medical history is the most important part of the history and will be covered in some detail.

1. Nature of dental anxiety

It is important from the outset to determine the nature of the patient's anxiety. Some people are anxious of 'dentistry' as a whole, whilst others have a specific anxiety about 'things in the mouth' or 'the dental drill' or 'dental injections' or 'having a tooth pulled'. The underlying basis for many of these anxiety-provoking stimuli is frequently the fear of 'pain'. Unfortunately, dentistry has always had a close association with pain and the possibility of pain-free dental treatment can be a very difficult concept for anxious patients to accept.

The extent of dental anxiety can range from mild apprehension to true phobia. Many phobic patients never actually make it to the surgery. Those who do, may present with poor dentition for routine conservation and are very different from the patient who has excellent dentition but is anxious about undergoing third molar surgery. It is important to try and gauge the degree of anxiety, and it can be useful to ask the patient about his or her fears and concerns about the dental visit.

This can help to break the ice and will steer the discussion in the right direction without unduly provoking sensitive emotions. In the case of fear of 'injections' or 'needles', the patient must be asked if this is a general fear or just specific to dentistry. Many patients have a fear of oral injections but will accept an injection in the arm. A true needle phobia will contraindicate the use of intravenous sedation without some form of premedication, topical anaesthetic agent or cognitive desensitisation therapy.

2. Dental history

A detailed knowledge of the past dental history is essential for planning dental treatment and determining suitability to receive treatment under sedation.

The dental history should ascertain details of why the patient is being considered for treatment under sedation. If the patient is dentally anxious then a history of when he or she first became anxious should be noted. For many patients this will have started with a bad experience in childhood but for others the onset of their anxiety may have been more recent, for example, following a traumatic extraction. Patients frequently state that they were quite happy to receive routine treatment until a specific dentist hurt them during treatment, which subsequently made them anxious about re-attending.

Information should also be sought about when (or even if) the patient last underwent routine dental treatment and the type of dentistry received. It is helpful to find out whether the patient has received sedation previously, what type of sedation this was and how they felt about it.

Finally, patients should be questioned regarding their concerns about their teeth, how they feel about their health and the appearance of their dentition, their future aspirations and any current dental symptoms. All of this information should then be compiled and used for treatment planning.

3. Medical history

The aim of medical history taking is to determine the fitness of the patient to undergo sedation and is the most important factor to consider during assessment. A full medical history should be taken in the same way as for any patient presenting for dental treatment but special note should be made of cardiovascular, respiratory, hepatic and renal disease. Full details of current drug therapy will alert the dentist to potential drug interactions and may reveal undisclosed conditions. Patients at the extremes of the age range, pregnant women and patients with disabilities and impairments deserve special consideration in relation to sedation. A medical history questionnaire may be helpful to ensure that all areas are covered and can provide prompts for further questioning.

Assessment of fitness for sedation

A useful means of estimating fitness for sedation is to use the classification system introduced by the American Society of Anesthesiologists (ASA). In this system patients are allocated to specific grades according to their medical status and operative (or sedation) risk. The classification uses six grades as follows:

ASA I   Normal healthy patients
ASA II   Patients with mild systemic disease
ASA III   Patients with severe systemic disease that is limiting but not incapacitating
ASA IV   Patients with incapacitating disease which is a constant threat to life
ASA V   Moribund patients not expected to live more than 24 hours

ASA I: Patients assessed as ASA class I are ideally suited to receive conscious sedation. They pose the lowest risk and can be safely treated in general dental practice. However, the possibility of undiagnosed medical problems should always be borne in mind, even in apparently healthy patients.

ASA II: ASA class II patients have a mild systemic disease. Examples might include well-controlled asthma, diet-controlled diabetes or mild hypertension. In addition to the true ASA II patients, it is also wise to include those who are extremely anxious about dental treatment. Extremely nervous patients have high circulating levels of endogenous adrenaline and are more prone to complications during sedation. Patients of ASA II present a higher risk but, with appropriate precautions, many are also suitable for treatment under sedation in dental practice.

ASA III: Individuals in ASA class III represent a group presenting a difficult choice as far as sedation is concerned. This group includes patients with, for example, stable angina, well-controlled epilepsy, chronic bronchitis, congestive heart failure or well-controlled insulin-dependent diabetes. These patients have a severe but controlled systemic disease, which may limit normal activity but which is not incapacitating. The use of sedation to reduce physiological and psychological stress can be very beneficial to this category of patients and may well reduce the risk of an acute exacerbation of the medical condition during dental treatment. However, such patients do present an increased risk and most of them should be referred to a specialist environment where extra support is available.

In addition to the true ASA III patients, it is also wise to include in this group patients who have no systemic disease, but who have a high body mass index (over 35) or are over 65 years of age. Patients who are significantly overweight may have a reduced respiratory capacity and older people are generally more sensitive to sedation agents and their physiological processes are slower.

ASA IV: ASA class IV represents patients who have severe life-threatening systemic disease. Examples include patients who have had a recent myocardial infarction, uncontrolled diabetes, uncontrolled epilepsy or severe emphysema requiring oxygen therapy. People in this category should usually be treated in an anaesthetist-led hospital day-stay facility where full medical and anaesthetic support is available.

ASA V: For patients in ASA class V, who are moribund, only emergency treatment would ever be provided. Such patients may be sedated for medical reasons but rarely for the purpose of providing dental treatment.

It is important to note that the ASA classification is not infallible, and there is some overlap between categories.

However, it does represent a relatively simple means of determining the risk of sedation. It is therefore essential to assess patients on an individual basis taking into consideration all elements of their medical and social history.

It can be difficult to classify patients with multiple conditions, e.g. a mildly asthmatic patient who has well-controlled diabetes. Where any condition falls into the higher ASA group this should be recorded as their physical status and the patient treated accordingly. In this way the risk to the patient is reduced and the dental treatment can be provided safely and effectively.

Relevance of specific medical conditions

To accurately assess and categorise the medical fitness of a patient for sedation, the dental clinician must have a clear understanding of specific pathological and physiological processes and their relevance to sedation practice.

Cardiovascular disease

Disease of the heart and circulatory system will affect a patient's fitness for treatment under sedation. In the Western world a high proportion of the population suffer from ischaemic heart disease and have a history of angina or a myocardial infarct. Other conditions such as valvular or congenital heart disease may also present to the dental clinician. In these patients the stress associated with dental treatment can lead to high levels of circulating adrenaline. This in turn causes tachycardia and hypertension, thereby increasing the load on the heart. When the cardiac status is already compromised stress may induce an acute exacerbation of the medical condition. The classic example of this would be the patient with stress-induced angina, who is at increased risk from acute myocardial infarction.

Hypertension resulting from vascular or renal disease affects many people, especially with increasing age. The stress of treatment and the effects of the sedation agent can cause significant fluctuations in blood pressure. Patients with a blood pressure below 160/95 should be able to receive sedation safely in dental practice. If the resting blood pressure is above this level, referral for medical evaluation before sedation is essential. In this regard, the diastolic reading is probably the more significant of the two values. As mentioned earlier, however, it is sudden changes in blood pressure that give rise to greater concern than the initial readings.

Although patients with cardiovascular disease benefit considerably from receiving treatment under sedation, they do present a special risk. Their limited ability to cope with stress increases the chance of an acute exacerbation of the disease during the sedation appointment. Many are also taking cardio-active medications which can interact with sedation agents.

Respiratory disease

Virtually all sedation agents cause some degree of respiratory depression, therefore good respiratory function is essential for patients undergoing sedation. Healthy patients with a normal respiratory capacity are able to compensate for the mild depressive effects of sedation drugs. However, patients with respiratory disease have less respiratory reserve and can easily become deoxygenated under sedation.

Asthma is a disease which is increasing in incidence, especially amongst children. Patients with well-controlled mild asthma can receive sedation in dental practice but it is important to be aware that the stress of treatment may make asthma worse and appropriate precautions should be taken. Asthmatic patients should be asked to take a dose of their normal bronchodilator, immediately before sedation and emergency drugs should be available in the case of an acute attack (see Chapter 8). If the asthma is severe, requiring oral steroids or hospitalisation, then the patient should be referred for sedation in an anaesthetist-led, hospital day-stay facility.

In chronic bronchitis and emphysema, respiratory capacity is also severely reduced and the stimulus to respiration can switch from a high carbon dioxide drive to a low oxygen drive. Caution should be exercised when considering sedation for this group of patients. Not only will the sedation agent cause further respiratory depression, but the use of supplemental oxygen is inadvisable as it may further inhibit respiratory drive and possibly cause hypnoea or apnoea. Such patients should not be managed in a primary care setting.

Upper respiratory tract infections, such as the common cold and sinusitis, present a relative contraindication to specific types of sedation. Inhalation sedation obviously requires a patent nasal airway for gas delivery but it is also important in intravenous sedation that the patient has no airway blockage. Chronic nasal obstruction caused by, for example, a deviated septum, is more problematic and inhalation techniques may prove impossible for physical reasons in such cases.

Hepatic and renal disorders

Liver and kidney diseases affect the metabolism and excretion of sedation drugs, especially those administered by the oral and intravenous routes. The normal pharmacokinetics of sedation agents are altered in hepatic and renal disease (see Chapter 2), and in patients with such conditions there can be a variable and unpredictable response. Those who receive sedation will be more sensitive to the sedative drug, may more easily become over-sedated and will take longer to recover. Any patient with a suspected history of hepatic or renal disease should be thoroughly investigated by a physician and, if the disease process is active or has resulted in permanent loss of function, intravenous and oral sedation should only be undertaken in an anaesthetist-led, hospital day-stay facility, following careful assessment.

Neurological disorders

There is a diverse range of conditions affecting the nervous system which can present problems with sedation. One of the most common conditions is epilepsy. Benzodiazepines, because of their anticonvulsant action, should reduce the incidence of an acute fit during treatment. However, sedation can mask the classical features of a grand mal seizure and if a convulsion does occur it may be difficult to diagnose. Unconsciousness may be the only sign, and the cause can be difficult to distinguish from other medical and sedation-related complications and emergencies. Sedation should be restricted for use in patients with well-controlled epilepsy and, where doubt exists, it should be undertaken in an anaesthetist-led, hospital day-stay facility where appropriate facilities are available to deal with an acute convulsion.

Endocrine disease

Diabetes, adrenal insufficiency and thyroid problems are the endocrine disorders which are most likely to cause problems in relation to sedation.

Diabetes: Diabetics who are diet-controlled or treated with oral hypoglycaemic drugs pose a minimal risk to sedation in dental practice. The main area of risk relates to type 1 diabetics (particularly when the diabetes is unstable and the blood sugar levels fluctuate significantly), where pre-operative starvation can upset the stability of blood sugar levels. Such patients should be managed with caution. Where the condition is well controlled the patient may be successfully treated under sedation provided the patient is scheduled for the first appointment of the morning. This allows them to have their breakfast and take their insulin as normal, maximising the stability of their condition. Where practical, inhalation sedation should be offered, as it is easily reversible in the event of a medical event. However, with careful assessment intravenous sedation may be used. Where the patient's diabetes is poorly controlled he/she should be referred to a secondary care facility for appropriate management and monitoring.

Adrenal insufficiency: Adrenal insufficiency can be potentially dangerous to a patient undergoing sedation. The response to stress is suppressed and there may be secondary hypertension or diabetes. Patients on long-term steroids may have similar problems as a result of adrenal suppression. These individuals are at considerable risk under sedation and should be referred to an anaesthetist-led, hospital day-stay facility where additional steroid cover can be given and full medical back up is available.

Thyroid disorders: Patients with thyroid disorders must be stabilised before undergoing sedation and any patient with active thyroid disease should always be referred to hospital. Hyperthyroidism can cause tachycardia or even atrial fibrillation, whilst hypothyroidism may produce bradycardia which can cause complications under sedation.

Haematological disorders

Anaemia is a common disorder which varies in severity. Mild anaemia, such as that occurring as a result of menstrual blood loss, does not present a problem to sedation in dental practice. However, sedation should be avoided in patients with a history of the more severe forms of anaemia, especially sickle cell anaemia and thalassaemia. Such patients are at severe risk if subjected to a reduced oxygen tension, which can occur during sedation as a result of respiratory depression, especially if the patient is over-sedated. The use of inhalation sedation in these patients may however be considered. It should also be noted that patients with anaemia are less likely to develop cyanosis due to the fact that they have less haemoglobin to become deoxygenated. Fortunately, this does not affect the readings of the pulse oximeter.

Disorders of the blood clotting system present a risk in relation to haemostasis. Injections should be avoided where at all possible and thus intravenous sedation is not the first method of choice for anxiolysis. Inhalation sedation with nitrous oxide is useful because it not only provides sedation but also produces some analgesia, which may obviate the need for dental local anaesthetic injections for simple conservative dentistry. A detailed history must be recorded for all patients with bleeding disorders or those who are receiving anticoagulant therapy and the advice of a haematologist sought, regarding the appropriateness of any dental treatment and its location.

![] ***Drug therapy***

Therapeutic drugs are intended to have a specific effect on one or more systems or organs of the body, but they can and frequently do produce coincidental side effects. Certain medicines interact with sedation drugs, so it is essential at the assessment visit to record accurately exactly what drugs a patient is taking and the diseases for which they have been prescribed. Each medicine must be checked for potential interaction with the proposed sedative agent to be used in the dental surgery. If the patient cannot remember which drugs have been prescribed, then the dental clinician must contact the patient's general medical practitioner for clarification prior to arranging care. It is essential to emphasise to patients undergoing sedation, that they should continue taking their normal medication, unless they have been told otherwise by their doctor.

Table 3.1 indicates some key groups of drugs which interact with the benzodiazepines. Some of the reactions are more theoretical possibilities and will depend on the duration and dosage of the prescribed medication. Care should always be taken, however, to ensure that a patient is not unnecessarily put at risk.

There are few absolute contraindications to sedation as a direct result of drug therapy. Normally the underlying medical

Table 3.1	Interactions of benzodiazepines with other drug groups
Drug	*Potential interaction*
Alcohol	enhanced sedative effect
Analgesics (opioid)	enhanced sedative effect
Antibacterials	erythromycin inhibits metabolism of midazolam
Antidepressants	enhanced sedative effect
Anti-epileptics	BDZs reduce effect of some antiepileptics
Anti-histamines	enhanced sedative effect
Anti-hypertensives	enhanced hypotensive effect
Anti-psychotics	enhanced sedative effect
Anti-ulcer drugs	cimetidine inhibits metabolosm of BDZs

condition will determine the ultimate fitness of a patient for treatment. If sedation is to go ahead then appropriate precautions must be taken to allow for potential drug interactions. If an enhanced sedative effect is expected, then the technique should be altered to slow the titration rate, reduce the total dose of sedation drug and allow more time for recovery.

Patients who are drug addicts or who abuse drugs should be considered with caution. Sedation may be difficult to achieve in these individuals and there are many unpredictable interactions that can occur with the recreational drugs. If there is any doubt about potential drug interaction then the patient should be referred to an anaesthetist-led, hospital day-stay facility for treatment.

Pregnancy

There are two main risks with providing sedation in pregnancy. First, the potential teratogenic and sedative effects of sedation drugs on the foetus. Second, the patient may have an atypical response to sedation as a result of altered metabolism from the additional demands of the foetus. For both of these reasons, it is preferable to postpone sedation until after the birth. Emergency or essential treatment should be undertaken in a hospital environment, preferably in the second trimester.

Intellectual or physical impairment

Patients with a learning disability present special problems. Sedation can help people with a mild learning disability undergo routine dental treatment whilst avoiding the need for reliance on general anaesthesia. Unfortunately the tolerance and response to sedation of those with a moderate or severe learning disability to is unpredictable and these patients are best managed in a specialist environment. In contrast, physically disabled patients usually respond very well to sedation and most patients can be treated in dental practice. The more severe physical disabilities will require the service of an anaesthetist-led, hospital day-stay service.

Age

Children and the elderly present a special risk to sedation, even if they are otherwise healthy. The metabolic rates of infants and young children are much higher than those of adults and their build is much smaller. The pharmacological effect of sedation agents in children is variable and if a complication occurs the child's condition can deteriorate very rapidly. Only inhalational sedation should be provided for children (under 16 years of age) in dental practice. Intravenous sedation with midazolam should only be carried out in children where inhalation sedation has either failed or is not indicated and only by those appropriately trained and experienced in administering paediatric intravenous sedation. Benzodiazepines, when administered to children, can produce disinhibition where the child becomes very confused and disorientated. This generally occurs where the child does not have a clear understanding of the effects of the sedation. It is therefore imperative when assessing a child for intravenous sedation, that consideration is given to the maturity of the child and his or her ability to manage the sedative effects.

In older people, the functioning of body systems becomes progressively less efficient. They are more susceptible to the effects of sedation agents with smaller doses are required to avoid over-sedation. There is an increased incidence of undiagnosed disease and elderly patients are less able to cope with undue stress. Although biological age rather than chronological age is the significant factor, caution should be exercised in sedating any patient over the age of 65.

If there is any doubt about a patient's medical status then communication with the general medical practitioner and/or referral to an anaesthetist-led, hospital day-stay facility for treatment is essential.

Importance of social circumstances

The final part of the history is to evaluate the domestic circumstances of the patient. A responsible adult will be required to accompany the patient to and from the surgery and the availability of suitable private transport is essential. It is important to ensure that the escort does not have additional responsibilities such as young children or elderly relatives. Adults should be questioned regarding their smoking habits, alcohol consumption and use of recreational drugs, as this may effect the action of the sedative agent used. General enquiries about their domestic circumstances should be made to ensure the patient will be safely cared for at home following treatment.

Clinical examination

Assessment of the patient for treatment under sedation should consist of a full clinical examination and an assessment of vital signs. Radiographs and other investigations should be obtained at the assessment visit and before the dental procedure whenever possible.

Oral exam

Some patients may allow a full oral examination, charting of the teeth and intra-oral radiography. Those presenting for specific oral surgical procedures will usually be amenable to a normal examination. However, patients with moderate to severe dental anxiety may only agree to a superficial visual inspection, without using a probe. If oral examination is not feasible the patient may instead be agreeable to extra-oral dental panoramic tomography.

The aim of the oral examination in anxious patients is to judge the type and extent of dental treatment required. This will help the dental clinician to determine whether the treatment can be performed under sedation, what is the most appropriate form of sedation, and to decide on the number of visits required. For the majority of anxious patients, who have often not been to a dentist for years, initial treatment will usually involve a gross scale, a number of extractions and routine conservation.

Sufficient information can usually be gleaned from which to compile a treatment plan for the first sedation appointment. Examination of anxious dental patients requires some degree of compromise, and occasionally full examination and intra-oral radiography will have to be postponed until a later date when the patient is sedated.

Assessment of vital signs

For all adult patients and those requiring dental treatment under intravenous sedation, it is essential at the assessment appointment to measure the heart rate, blood pressure, respiration rate, arterial oxygen saturation level, weight and height. The purpose of taking preliminary values is threefold:
  (i)   to determine the patient's fitness for sedation
  (ii) to provide baselines for comparison with future measurements taken during sedation
  (iii) as a screening to reveal possible undiagnosed disease.

Blood pressure and heart rate

Some degree of elevation in the cardio-respiratory signs, such as tachycardia or systolic hypertension, above the normal range for the age and sex of the patient, is to be expected at the assessment appointment. This is caused by acute apprehension felt by anxious dental patients when they attend the dental surgery.

Blood pressure can be measured using either a manual or automatic sphygmomanometer. The blood pressure can be

Table 3.2	Blood pressure values and associated ASA class
Blood pressure	*ASA class*
Less than 140/90	I
From 140/90 to 159/94	II
From 160/95 to 199/114	III
Over 200/115	IV

used to categorise a patient into an appropriate ASA class as shown in Table 3.2 (based on Malamed, 1997).

As previously stated, patients with a blood pressure below 160/95 can be treated under sedation in dental practice. If the blood pressure is above this level patients should be referred to their general medical practitioner for full evaluation before considering sedation.

Oxygen saturation

Using a pulse oximeter, arterial oxygen saturation can be monitored, providing a record of the patient's respiratory function. Average oxygen saturation values are 97% to 99% in the healthy individual. An oxygen saturation value of 95% may be clinically accepted in a patient with a normal haemoglobin level.

Body mass index

Body mass index (BMI) relates a person's body weight to height. The BMI is a person's weight in kilograms (kg) divided by their height in metres squared (m²). A BMI of 18.5–24.9 is considered to be an ideal height to weight ratio for an adult; below 18.5 is defined as underweight. Overweight is defined as a BMI of 25–29.9 and obesity as a BMI of 30 and above. Note, however, that some very muscular people may have a high BMI without undue health risks.

Patients who are obese should be treated with caution. If the BMI is greater than 35, the patient will not be suitable for intravenous sedation in dental practice as they are more at risk of respiratory and cardiovascular complications. These patients should be referred to an anaesthetist-led, hospital day-stay facility. The patient may be treated more safely under inhalation sedation in a dental practice setting, and this should be considered at the assessment stage. At the other end of the spectrum, patients who have a very small build, especially children and the elderly, tend to be more susceptible to the effects of sedation.

Treatment planning

Armed with the detailed information from the history and examination, a preliminary treatment plan can now be established. This needs to specify both the type of sedation or anaesthesia plus the dental treatment required. It needs to be approached logically and flexibly, allowing for modifications if they become necessary.

Choice of sedation technique

Although this chapter has focused on assessing the suitability of patients for sedation, it is important to remember the range of treatment options, including:
  (i)   Local analgesia alone
 (ii)   Sedation and local analgesia
(iii)   General anaesthesia.

In considering the type of sedation or anaesthesia, account should be taken of the patient's medical fitness, social circumstances, degree of anxiety and expected level of co-operation, plus the extent and duration of the planned dental treatment. It is also important to establish the clinical need for the type of sedation or anaesthesia selected. Some patients, such as those with minimal anxiety requiring relatively simple surgical extractions, may be agreeable to having treatment under local analgesia alone. Others may be so terrified because of their phobia, lack adequate co-operation or require traumatic or extensive dental procedures that general anaesthesia would be the best choice. In between these two extremes there is a large proportion of patients for whom techniques of pharmacological sedation represents the most acceptable means of undergoing dental treatment.

   Careful explanation and discussion of the different types of sedation with the patient is essential. The dental clinician should describe the main features of oral, inhalation and intravenous techniques and point out the key differences between sedation and general anaesthesia. Many patients have the preconceived idea that they will only undergo treatment if they are completely 'asleep' or 'knocked out completely'. It is important to explain that sedation produces relaxation, decreased awareness and often amnesia, but not unconsciousness. Reassurance should also be given about painless local anaesthetic administration and the use of topical analgesia.

All explanations must be carried out in a particularly considerate manner and the patient's reaction during the explanation is helpful in deciding the most appropriate sedation technique. Patients should also be reassured that they remain in control of their own destiny and that no treatment will be forced upon them against their wishes (see Chapter 10).

Dental treatment plan

The treatment plan depends on a number of factors. The patient's current dental condition, predicted future attendance pattern and compliance with oral health instructions should all be taken into account. The purpose of this is to provide good quality dentistry consistent with the patient's realistic aspirations. There is little point in doing molar endodontics or bridgework in a patient who is unlikely to maintain their oral health in the long term.

Treatment of teeth that are causing symptoms should be the first priority. This will be followed by extraction of retained roots and grossly carious or periodontally-involved teeth. Gross scaling and simple, good quality conservation should be the mainstay of treatment for the remaining teeth. These are only general recommendations and it is essential that each patient has a tailored individual treatment plan. The patient should be given an estimate of the number of appointments that will be required to complete the work and of the arrangements for long-term follow up.

Preparation of patients for sedation

Patients who are scheduled to receive sedation must receive careful spoken and written instructions (Figure 3.1) as to their responsibilities before and after the sedation appointment.

For oral and intravenous sedation, the patient should be accompanied by a responsible adult. With inhalation sedation for adults, this is a slightly controversial subject, since there is good evidence that patients acquire their normal faculties within minutes of sedation being terminated. However, an escort is still recommended. Escorts must accompany the patient to and from the dental practice and must assume responsibility for the patient's post-sedation care. Wherever possible the patient and escort should travel home by private car or taxi rather than by public transport. Patients should be warned against driving, operating machinery (including domestic appliances), drinking alcohol, signing legal documents or undertaking Internet transactions for a period of 24 hours following sedation.

SEDATION DEPARTMENT
APPOINTMENT FOR SEDATION

Name: ……………………………… Hospital No: ……………………..

An appointment has been made for you to attend the Sedation Department on:
……………………………………………………………………. At ………………………………..

If you are unable to keep this appointment please telephone the department as soon as possible on…………………………….

INSTRUCTION FOR PATIENTS HAVING TREATMENT UNDER SEDATION

You have been given an appointment for dental treatment under sedation. It is important you observe the following instructions or your treatment may have to be postponed:

1. You MUST NOT eat or drink anything for two hours prior to your appointment time. Before this you should have a light meal, e.g. toast and tea, coffee or fruit juice.

2. No alcohol is to be consumed 24 hours prior to the appointment.

3. You must be accompanied by a responsible adult who must be present in the waiting area at the beginning of your appointment. He/she must remain in the building throughout the appointment, escort you home afterwards and arrange for you to be looked after for the following 24 hours. The accompanying adult must not be in charge of any people, adults or children, other than the patient.

4. If you are taking any medicines they should be taken at the usual times and should also be brought with you to the clinic.

5. Any illnesses occurring before the appointment should be reported immediately, as this may affect your treatment.

6. Ensure nail varnish and false nails are removed before the appointment.

7. Your escort should take you home after treatment by private car or taxi and NOT public transport.

8. You MUST NOT drive any vehicle, operate machinery, use any domestic appliance or use the Internet for 24 hours following sedation.

9. You MUST NOT drink alcohol, return to work, make any important decisions or sign any legal documents for 24 hours after sedation.

10. You are advised to leave any valuables with the person accompanying you, or at home. No responsibility can be taken for any valuables lost on the Sedation Department premises.

If you follow these instructions you should have a pleasant and uneventful recovery from your treatment under sedation. Please feel free at any time to ask the sedation nurse or clinician any questions that you may have about your treatment.

Figure 3.1 Written instruction sheet for patients scheduled for treatment under sedation.

It is recommended that patients are asked to starve for a period of 2 hours before the sedation appointment. However within 2–4 hours of sedation, patients should be advised to take a light meal with tea or fruit juice. Longer periods of starvation are not advisable, as the relative hypoglycaemia that occurs during starvation may precipitate fainting during the sedation appointment. Additionally, long periods of starvation result in acid build-up in the stomach and the risk of regurgitation rises. In an appropriately sedated patient the protective laryngeal reflexes are not obtunded and thus the risk of aspiration if the patient vomits should be minimal.

Consent

Written, informed consent must be obtained from all patients who are to receive treatment under sedation. The dental clinician must carefully explain to the patient what to expect at the treatment appointment. This should include a description of the sedation technique and its side effects and details of the dentistry to be provided, as well as any viable alternatives. The patient should sign a consent form giving permission for the sedation, the local analgesia and dental treatment. It is not best practice to leave obtaining consent until the day of treatment, when the patient may be particularly anxious and unable to make clear judgements for valid consent. Equally, however, consent should be obtained within a reasonable period of time prior to the appointment for sedation. (It should also be reconfirmed on the day of treatment.) Finally, any remaining questions that the patient has should be answered and an appointment should then be made to start treatment under sedation.

Assessment record

Full details of the history, examination and treatment plan must be recorded in the patient notes. It is also useful to complete a sedation assessment form, an example of which is shown in Figure 3.2. Use of a standardised form ensures that all aspects of the assessment are covered and also provides a readily accessible summary which can be referred to at the treatment appointment. If all the documentation is correctly completed, the likelihood of accidents is reduced and the defence of any accusations facilitated.

Affix patient identification label in box below or complete details	
Surname	Patient ID No.
Forename	D.O.B. D D M M Y Y Y Y
Address	NHS No.
	Sex. Male / Female
Postcode	

SEDATION ASSESSMENT

Assessment Date	Assessed by

Social History	Relevant Details
Age/Occupation Smoking/Alcohol	

Medical Conditions	Relevant Details
Cardiovascular disease	
Respiratory disease	
Hepatic/Renal disease	
Bleeding/Epilepsy/Diabetes	
Anaemia/Jaundice/Hepatitis	
Other Serious Illness	
Operation/GA/Sedation	
Drug Therapy	
Drugs/Medication	
Allergies	

Vital Signs						**ASA Class**
Weight (kg)	Height (m)	BMI (kg/m^2)	Blood pressure	Pulse	Respiration Rate	

Treatment Plan	
Type of Sedation	Intravenous Inhalational Oral
Fulfil criteria for OP Sedation?	YES/NO If NO refer for in-patient care
Dental treatment plan -1 -2 -3	
Written consent	
Written information/instructions	
Waiting List	

Clinician Signature	

Figure 3.2 Sedation assessment record.

References and further reading

Malamed, S.F. (1995) *Sedation: A Guide to Patient Management.*
    St Louis, Mosby: pp 32–62.
Malamed, S.F. (2007) *Medical Emergencies in the Dental Office.*
    St Louis, Mosby.
Royal College of Surgeons of England (1993) *Guidelines for Sedation by
    Non-anaesthetists.* Report of a working party. London, RCSEng.

4 Pharmacology of inhalation and intravenous sedation

▓▓▓▓ INTRODUCTION

A sound understanding of the principles of the phamacology of the individual sedation agents is essential to the safe practice of sedation. It is important from the outset to specify exactly what is meant by a sedation agent, as there can be considerable overlap between drugs which produce both sedation and general anaesthesia. A drug used for sedation should:
1. Depress the central nervous system (CNS) to an extent that allows operative treatment to be carried out with minimal physiological and psychological stress
2. Modify the patient's state of mind such that communication is maintained and the patient will respond to spoken command
3. Carry a margin of safety wide enough to render the unintended loss of consciousness and loss of protective reflexes unlikely.

Current sedation practice should only use agents and techniques which satisfy the above criteria. Additionally, the agents themselves should have a:
1. Simple method of administration
2. Rapid onset
3. Predictable action and duration
4. Rapid recovery
5. Rapid metabolism and excretion
6. Low incidence of side effects.

Sedation agents are usually administered via the inhalation, intravenous or oral routes. The route of administration affects the timing of drug action, although ultimately all drugs arrive at their target cells in the brain via the bloodstream.

Inhalation agents have the advantage of being readily absorbed by the lungs to provide a rapid onset of sedation, followed by rapid elimination and recovery. Intravenous agents are predictably absorbed but once administered cannot be removed from the bloodstream. The therapeutic action of intravenous agents is terminated by re-distribution, metabolism and excretion. Oral sedatives have a less certain absorption due to variability of gastric emptying and they therefore produce unpredictable levels of sedation.

This chapter will primarily address the pharmacology of sedation agents currently used in inhalation and intravenous techniques. The pharmacology of the oral sedatives not included in this chapter, will be covered in Chapter 5.

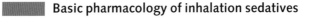 INHALATION SEDATION AGENTS

Inhalation agents produce sedation by their action on various areas of the brain. They reach the brain by entering the lungs, crossing the alveolar membrane into the pulmonary veins, returning with the blood to the left side of the heart and then passing into the systemic arterial circulation. Thus the two main components of inhalation sedation are, the entry of the inspired gas into the lungs and distribution of the agent by the circulation to the tissues.

Basic pharmacology of inhalation sedatives

Gas solubility and partial pressure

During the induction of inhalation sedation, each breath of sedation agent raises the partial pressure of the gas in the alveoli. As the alveolar partial pressure rises, the gas is forced across the alveolar membrane into the bloodstream, where it is carried to the site of action in the brain. The gas passes down a pressure gradient from areas of high partial pressure to areas of low partial pressure (Figure 4.1). The level of sedation is proportional to the partial pressure of the agent at the site of action. After termination of gas administration the reverse process occurs. The partial pressure in the alveoli falls and the gas passes in the opposite direction out of the brain, into the circulation and then into the lungs.

The rate at which a gas passes down its pressure gradient is determined by its solubility. The solubility of a sedation agent (i.e. the blood-gas partition coefficient) determines how quickly the partial pressure in the blood and, ultimately the brain, will rise or fall. The higher the partition coefficient, the greater the alveolar concentration of the agent needs to be to produce a rise in partial pressure in the blood and ultimately the tissues.

For the purposes of sedation, a gas with a low partition coefficient is preferred. Small concentrations of gas will

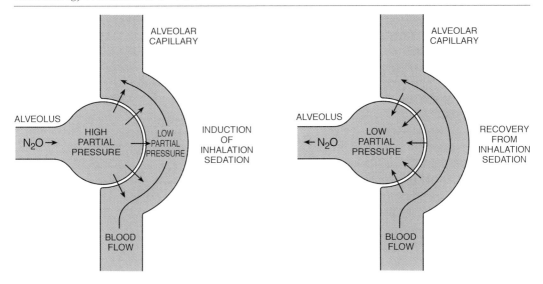

produce a rapid rise in partial pressure and a fast onset of sedation. Similarly, after cessation of gas administration there will be a rapid fall in partial pressure and a fast recovery.

It is the inspired concentration of sedation agent which will determine the final level of sedation. The speed of induction of sedation is influenced by the rate of increase in gas concentration, as well as the minute volume and cardiac output of the patient. Any increase in minute volume, such as can be caused by asking the patient to take deep breaths, will increase the speed of onset of sedation.

Conversely, an increase in cardiac output will reduce the speed of induction of sedation. With a high cardiac output there is an increased volume of blood passing through the lungs. The sedation agent present in the lungs will be taken up into this larger volume of blood and the actual concentration of gas transported per unit volume of blood will be lower. Thus, less sedation agent will reach the brain and there will be a slower onset of sedation. The speed of recovery after termination of gas administration is similarly affected by the same factors.

Potency of inhalation sedation agents

All sedation agents will produce general anaesthesia if used in high enough doses. The key to modern sedation practice is to ensure that the agents used have a wide enough margin of safety to render the unintended loss of consciousness unlikely. This means that there should be a considerable difference in the dose required to produce a state of sedation and the dose needed to induce general anaesthesia.

Figure 4.1
Movement of nitrous oxide gas down the partial pressure gradient during induction and recovery from inhalational sedation.

For inhalation anaesthetic agents the potency is expressed in terms of a minimum alveolar concentration (MAC). The MAC of an agent is the inspired concentration which will, at equilibrium, abolish the response to a standard surgical stimulus in 50% of patients.

Although the inspired concentration is measured as a percentage, the MAC is usually expressed as a number. Equilibrium is achieved when the tissue concentration of the gas equals the inspired concentration. MAC is a useful index of potency and is used to compare different anaesthetic gases.

Gases used for sedation should preferably have a moderate or high MAC and a low solubility. This will ensure a broad margin of safety between the incremental doses used to produce sedation and the final concentration required to induce anaesthesia. It would be very easy, using an agent with a small MAC for sedation, to accidentally overdose and anaesthetise a patient.

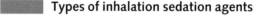

Types of inhalation sedation agents

Nitrous oxide

Nitrous oxide is the only inhalation agent currently in routine use for conscious sedation in dental practice. It was discovered by Joseph Priestly in 1772 and first used as an anaesthetic agent for dental exodontia by Horace Wells in 1844. Nitrous oxide has been used as the basic constituent of gaseous anaesthesia for the subsequent 160 years, demonstrating its acceptability and usefulness. In the 1930s, nitrous oxide was used for sedation purposes in the Scandinavian countries, particularly Denmark. However, it was not until the 1960s, when Harold Langa pioneered the modern practice of relative analgesia that nitrous oxide came into widespread use as an inhalation sedation agent in dentistry.

Presentation: Nitrous oxide is a colourless, faintly sweet-smelling gas with a specific gravity of 1.53. It is stored in light blue cylinders in liquid form at a pressure of 750 pounds per square inch (43.5 bar).

The gas is sold by weight and each cylinder is stamped with its empty weight. As the contents of the cylinder are liquid, the pressure inside, as measured by the pressure gauge on the inhalational sedation machine, will remain constant until nearly all the liquid has evaporated. The value shown on the gauge does not decrease in a linear fashion and tends to fall rapidly immediately before the cylinder becomes empty (Figure 4.2).

Thus, the only reliable means of assessing the amount of nitrous oxide in a cylinder is to weigh the cylinder and compare the value with the weight of the empty cylinder. It can also be

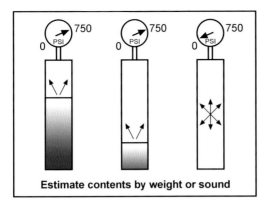

Estimate contents by weight or sound

Figure 4.2
The pressure in the nitrous oxide cylinder remains constant and tends to fall rapidly immediately before the cylinder becomes empty.

tapped with a metal instrument by those with musical ears; the pitch of the note falls as the gas is used. In addition, after prolonged use, the evaporation of the liquid nitrous oxide causes ice crystallisation on the cylinder at the level of the liquid within, thereby providing a third indication as to the nitrous oxide volume remaining in the cylinder.

***Blood/gas solubility*:** Nitrous oxide has a low blood-gas partition coefficient of 0.47, so it is relatively insoluble and produces rapid induction of sedation. A further consequence of the poor solubility is that, when administration is discontinued, nitrous oxide dissolved in the blood is rapidly eliminated via the lungs. During the first few minutes of this elimination, large volumes of nitrous oxide pour out of the blood and into the lungs. This can actually displace oxygen from the alveoli causing a condition known as *diffusion hypoxia*. This occurs because the volume of nitrous oxide in the alveoli is so high that the patient effectively 'breathes' 100% nitrous oxide. For this reason the patient should receive 100% oxygen for a period of at least 2–3 minutes after the termination of nitrous oxide sedation. In reality, the risk of diffusion hypoxia is minimal due to the high level of oxygen delivered by dedicated inhalation sedation machines.

***Potency*:** Nitrous oxide has a theoretical minimum alveolar concentration (MAC) of about 110. The high MAC means that nitrous oxide is a weak anaesthetic which is readily titrated to produce sedation. Because the MAC is over 80, it is theoretically impossible to produce anaesthesia using nitrous oxide alone, at normal atmospheric pressure, in a patient who is adequately oxygenated. However, caution should be exercised when using inhaled concentrations of nitrous oxide over 50%, because even at this relatively low percentage, some patients may enter a stage of light anaesthesia.

***Sedation*:** Nitrous oxide is a good, but mild sedation agent producing both a depressant and euphoriant effect on the CNS.

It is also a fairly potent analgesic. A 50% inhaled concentration of nitrous oxide has been equated to that of parenteral morphine injection at a standard dose (10mg in a 70kg adult). It can be used to good effect to facilitate simple dentistry in patients who are averse to local analgesia and it decreases the pain of injections in those who require supplemental local anaesthesia. Nitrous oxide has few side effects in therapeutic use. It causes minor cardio-respiratory depression, and produces no useful amnesia.

Occupational hazards of nitrous oxide: The main problems associated with the use of nitrous oxide relate not to the patient but to the staff providing sedation, and the potential hazards of chronic exposure to nitrous oxide gas have recently been recognised. It has been shown that regular exposure of healthcare personnel to nitrous oxide can cause specific illnesses, the most common effects being haematological disorders and reproductive problems (Figure 4.3).

Figure 4.3
Hazards of chronic exposure to nitrous oxide.

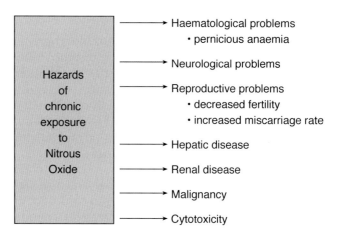

It is well known that nitrous oxide causes the oxidation of vitamin B12 and affects the functioning of the enzyme methionine synthetase. This in turn impairs haematopoesis and can give rise to pernicious anaemia in staff exposed to nitrous oxide for prolonged periods (Figure 4.4).

Dental clinicians who have abused nitrous oxide have been shown to have the debilitating neurological signs of pernicious anaemia. It has been shown that where unscavenged nitrous oxide has been used, there may be an increase in the rate of miscarriages in female dental surgeons, dental nurses and, perhaps surprisingly, in the wives of male dental surgeons who have been exposed to nitrous oxide gas. Dental nurses assisting with nitrous oxide sedation, where scavenging is not provided, are also twice as likely to suffer a miscarriage as other dental

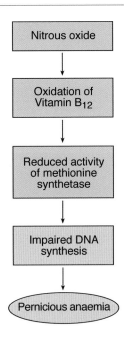

Figure 4.4
Biochemical effect of chronic nitrous oxide exposure.

nurses. Chronic exposure to nitrous oxide has also been shown to be associated with decreased female and male fertility. Other chronic effects of nitrous oxide exposure are much rarer but are said to include hepatic and renal disease, malignancy and cytotoxicity.

It should be noted that it is the cumulative effect of the gas which is the major concern and that the effects of the nitrous oxide very much depend on:
1. The pattern of exposure
2. Tissue sensitivity
3. Vitamin B12 intake and body stores
4. Extent to which methionine synthetase is deactivated.

The subject of nitrous oxide pollution has become a worldwide health and safety issue, particularly as it is described as a 'greenhouse gas' and appears to contribute to the damage of the ozone layer. Regulations have therefore been put in place to define the maximum acceptable occupational exposure of personnel to nitrous oxide. In the UK, exposure should not average more than 100 ppm over an 8-hour period under the current health and safety regulations. Since the initial studies into the effects of chronic exposure in healthcare personnel working with nitrous oxide, the risks have been reduced considerably by the introduction of efficient scavenging and ventilation systems. If exhaled nitrous oxide is actively removed there will be less pollution of the atmosphere where healthcare personnel are working. Better training and understanding of the technique has also led to more efficient and effective provision of inhalation sedation.

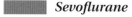 *Sevoflurane*

Sevoflurane is receiving much attention in the field of sedation research as a possible agent for use in dentistry. It is a sweet-smelling, non-flammable, volatile anaesthetic agent used for induction and maintenance of general anaesthesia. Sevoflurane is a potent agent with a MAC value of under 2, leaving it with a narrow margin of safety. Its use in sedation necessitates the use of a specialised vapouriser to ensure levels are kept to a subanaesthetic level of 0.3%. Other volatile anaesthetic agents such as halothane and isoflurane have also been tested for use in inhalational sedation. Unfortunately they are even more potent drugs than sevoflurane, with low MAC values (the MAC of halothane is 0.76). This again reduces the margin of safety and makes the induction of general anaesthesia more likely. These drugs are not currently suitable for providing sedation in dental practice and do not comply with the basic definitions of safe sedation, however research into the use of sevoflurane is promising.

Oxygen

Oxygen is not a sedation agent, however, inhalation sedation agents are always delivered in an oxygen-rich mixture containing a minimum of 30% oxygen by volume. Oxygen is stored as a gas in black cylinders with white shoulders, at an initial pressure of 2000 pounds per square inch (137 bar).

Because it is a gas under pressure, the gauge on the inhalational sedation machine will give an accurate representation of the amount of oxygen contained in the cylinder. The oxygen supply used for inhalational sedation should be separate from, and additional to, the supply kept for use in the management of emergencies. Oxygen will sustain and enhance combustion and therefore no naked flames should be allowed in an area where oxygen is being used.

INTRAVENOUS SEDATION AGENTS

Intravenous sedation agents are injected directly into the bloodstream where they are carried in the plasma to the tissues. The plasma level of the sedative attained during injection causes the agent to diffuse down its concentration gradient and across the lipid membranes to the site of action in the brain. The factors which influence the plasma level of the drug are therefore instrumental in determining the onset of action and recovery from the effect of the sedation agent.

 BASIC PHARMACOLOGY OF INTRAVENOUS SEDATIVES

 Induction of sedation

Upon intravenous injection the plasma level of a sedation drug will rise rapidly. The agent will pass through the venous system to the right side of the heart and then via the pulmonary circulation to the left side of the heart. Once in the arterial system it will reach the brain but it will only start to have its effect once diffusion across the lipid membranes has occurred. The effect of sedation will normally commence in one arm-brain circulation time, approximately 35 seconds. The final plasma concentration of the sedation agent will depend on the total dose of drug, the rate of the injection, the cardiac output and the circulating blood volume. The greater the dose of drug injected and the faster the rate of injection then the higher the plasma concentration. In contrast, the higher the cardiac output and/or the blood volume, the lower the plasma concentration.

 Recovery from sedation

Recovery from sedation occurs by two processes. The first is the redistribution of the sedation agent from the CNS into the body fat. The initial peak plasma concentration forces the sedation agent into tissues which are well-perfused such as the brain, heart, liver and kidneys. With time, an increasing amount of the sedation agent is taken into adipose tissue. Although solubility in fat is lower than in well-perfused tissues, the high mass of the body fat and the lipid solubility of sedation agents does promote redistribution to the fat stores. Ultimately the plasma concentration of drug falls and the blood-brain concentration gradient is reversed. This forces the sedation agent out of the brain and back into the bloodstream. The second process involves the uptake and metabolism of the sedation agent in the liver and elimination via the kidneys. This results in the final reduction in plasma concentration leading to complete recovery of the patient.

The relative importance of redistribution and elimination depends on the individual sedation agent but in general, redistribution is responsible for the initial recovery from sedation (the alpha half-life; $T_{1/2}\alpha$), followed by elimination of the remaining drug (the beta half-life; $T_{1/2}\beta$). Virtually all intravenous agents have two half-lives. Only those with very rapid metabolism do not demonstrate a bi-phasic curve. In considering different drugs, however, it is the elimination half-life which can be used to compare the pharmacokinetic effects of different sedation agents.

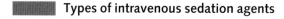 ## Types of intravenous sedation agents

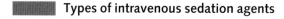 ### *Benzodiazepines*

It was not until the 1960s that agents were developed specifically for conscious sedation. At this time a group of tranquilising drugs known as the benzodiazepines were discovered in Switzerland by researchers at Hoffman-La Roche. Since then the benzodiazepines have become the mainstay of modern sedation practice in the United Kingdom. The first benzodiazepine to come on the market was diazepam (Valium®). Since then, other drugs including midazolam and temazepam have been developed which are used in the field of dental sedation.

Pharmacokinetics: To understand the mechanism of action of the benzodiazepines, it is necessary to appreciate the normal passage of information through sensory neurones to the CNS. A system made up of 'GABA' (gamma-amino-butyric-acid) receptors is responsible for filtering or damping down sensory input to the brain. GABA is an inhibitory chemical which is released from sensory nerve endings as electrical nerve stimuli pass from neurone to neurone over synapses. Once released, GABA attaches itself to receptors on the cell membrane of the post-synaptic neurone. The post-synaptic membrane becomes more permeable to chloride ions which has the effect of stabilising the neurone and increasing the threshold for firing (Figure 4.5).

During this refractory period no further electrical stimuli can be transmitted across the synapse. In this way the numbers of sensory messages which travel the whole distance of the neurones (from their origin to the areas of the brain where they are perceived) are reduced or 'filtered'. For every stimulus to the senses (touch, taste, smell, hearing, sight), very many more electrical stimuli are initiated than are necessary for the subject to perceive the stimulus and react to it.

Benzodiazepines act throughout the CNS via the GABA network. Specific benzodiazepine receptors are located close to GABA receptors on neuronal membranes within the brain and spinal cord. All benzodiazepines (which, like all sedatives, are CNS depressants) have a similar shape, with a ring structure (benzene ring) on the same position of the diazepine part of each molecule. It is this common core shape which enables

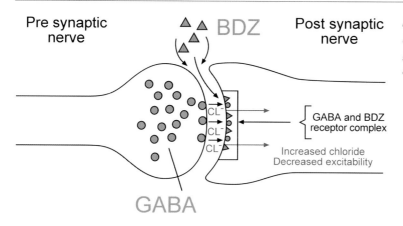

Figure 4.5
Mechanism of action of gamma-aminobutyric acid (GABA).

them to attach to the benzodiazepine receptors. The effect of having a benzodiazepine in place on a receptor, is to prolong the time it takes for re-polarisation after a neurone has been depolarised by an electrical impulse. This further reduces the number of stimuli reaching the higher centres and produces pharmacological sedation, anxiolysis, amnesia, muscle relaxation and anticonvulsant effects. Benzodiazepines act essentially by mimicking the normal physiological filter system of the body and they may do so positively or negatively.

There is a range of benzodiazepines which vary from those having the desired effects (agonists), to those having the entirely opposite effect (inverse agonists). In the centre of the spectrum is a group of drugs which have an affinity for the benzodiazepine receptor but which are, to all intents and purposes, pharmacologically inactive (antagonists).

Clinical effects: The clinical effects of the agonist benzodiazepines include:

- Induction of a state of conscious sedation with acute detachment for 20–30 minutes and a state of relaxation for a further hour or so
- Production of anterograde amnesia (loss of memory in the period immediately following the introduction of the drug)
- Muscle relaxation
- Anticonvulsant action
- Minimal cardiovascular and respiratory depression when intravenous benzodiazepines are titrated slowly to a defined end point of conscious sedation in healthy patients. (Titration refers to the process of adding small increments of a sedative whilst observing the clinical response until it is deemed adequate)

Benzodiazepines do not produce any clinically useful analgesia, although the sedation itself may alter the patient's response to pain.

Side effects: Although intravenous benzodiazepines are generally very safe sedation agents, they do have some disadvantages, including:
- Respiratory depression
- Cardiovascular depression
- Over-sedation in older people and children
- Tolerance
- Sexual fantasy.

The most significant side effect is respiratory depression. Some degree of respiratory depression occurs in all patients sedated with the benzodiazepines but this usually only becomes clinically significant in patients with impaired respiratory function or in those who have taken other CNS depressants or where the drug is administered too rapidly or in a bolus dose .

Pre-existing respiratory disease: A patient with pre-existing respiratory disease will already have a degree of respiratory compromise and will be especially at risk from the respiratory depressant effects of the benzodiazepines.

Synergistic effect: There is a synergistic relationship between the benzodiazepines and certain other CNS depressants, such as the opiates or alcohol. In a synergistic relationship, the effect of two drugs is greater than the sum total of the individual drugs and this is particularly noticeable with the opiates, when required doses may be 25% or less than if a single drug had been administered. The risk, therefore, of overdose in combined drug techniques is significantly higher than when a single agent is used.

Inappropriate drug administration: Excessively rapid intravenous injection of the benzodiazepines can cause significant respiratory depression which may result in apnoea. This can be avoided by slow incremental injection of the drug. If apnoea does occur, then assisted ventilation will be required. It is also thought that the laryngeal reflexes may be momentarily obtunded immediately following injection of a benzodiazepine. Although this state is short-lived, the dental clinician should always ensure that the patient's airway is well protected when performing dental treatment on sedated patients.

Because of the risk of apnoea, it has been suggested by some authorities that supplemental oxygen be used in all patients. However, this is not universally practised and it is questionable as to whether it is really indicated in fit, young healthy patients. There is little doubt, however, that supplemental oxygen does result in the maintenance of better oxygen saturation and it should, therefore, be considered in cases where appropriate, particularly in older or medically compromised patients.

The benzodiazepines also produce minor cardiovascular side effects in healthy patients. They cause a reduction in vascular resistance which results in a fall in blood pressure. This is compensated by an increase in heart rate, and the cardiac output and usually blood pressure are thus unaffected.

Older patients are particularly susceptible to the effects of the benzodiazepines. It is relatively easy to overdose an older patient and cause significant respiratory depression. Intravenous benzodiazepines should be administered slowly and in very small increments to older people. The total dose required to produce sedation will be much smaller than in a younger adult of the equivalent weight. The use of intravenous benzodiazepines for children under the age of 16 years in a primary care setting should be considered carefully. Children may react more unpredictably to intravenous benzodiazepines and can easily become over-sedated. Occasionally they may show signs of disinhibition and become extremely distraught, a reaction more common in the teenage years. Extreme care needs to be undertaken with such patients, as the temptation to keep adding further increments can easily result in an unconscious patient. Treating children under intravenous benzodiazepine sedation requires that the dental clinician is appropriately trained in the use of this technique and is fully competent in the provision of paediatric basic life support.

Patients who are already taking oral benzodiazepines for anxiolysis or insomnia may be tolerant to the effect of intravenous benzodiazepines. Those who have become dependant on long-term benzodiazepine therapy may also have their dependence reactivated by acute intravenous administration.

There have also been reported incidents of sexual fantasy occurring under intravenous benzodiazepine sedation but this only seems to occur when higher than recommended doses of the drug are administered.

Diazepam

Diazepam was the first benzodiazepine to be used in intravenous sedation practice (see Figure 4.6). It is almost insoluble in water and so it is either dissolved in an organic solvent, propylene glycol (Valium®), or it is emulsified into a suspension in soya bean oil (Diazemuls®). The organic solvent formulation caused a high incidence of vein damage, ranging from pain to frank thrombophlebitis and even skin ulceration, so this preparation is no longer used. Diazemuls® is a non-irritant preparation which overcomes the problem of venous damage.

Diazepam is metabolised in the liver and eliminated via the kidneys. It has a long elimination half-life ($T_{1/2}\beta$) of 43 hours

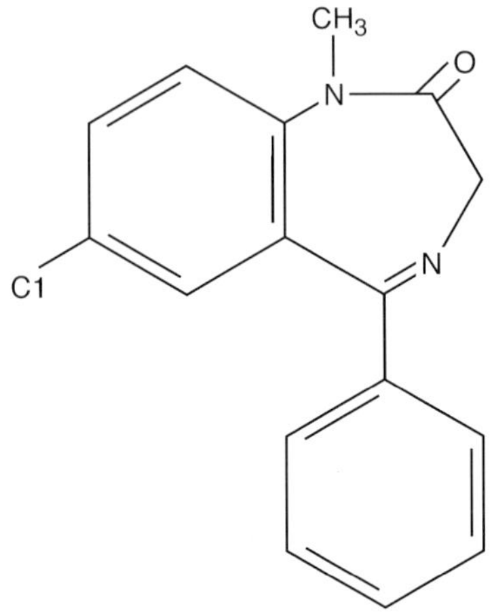

Figure 4.6
Chemical structure of
diazepam, showing a
benzene ring structure
attached to the diazepine
part of the molecule.

Diazepam

(+/−13 hours) although its distribution half-life (T1/2α) is in the
region of 40 minutes. An active metabolite, n-desmethyldiazepam,
is produced, which can cause rebound sedation up to 72 hours
after the initial administration of diazepam.

Diazemuls® is presented in a 2ml ampoule in a
concentration of 5mg/ml for intravenous injection. It is a
reliable hypnosedative which should be given slowly, titrating
the dose against the response obtained. The standard dose lies
in the range 0.1-0.2mg/kg. Unfortunately the long recovery
period and possibility of rebound sedation mean that diazepam
in any form, is not the ideal drug for sedation for short dental
procedures and its use has largely been superseded by the
more modern and more rapidly metabolised midazolam.

Midazolam

Midazolam was introduced into clinical practice in 1983
although it had been synthesised several years previously (see
Figure 4.7). It is currently the agent of choice for intravenous
sedation in dentistry, however there are newer agents on the
horizon.

It is an imadazobenzodiazepine which is water soluble with
a pH of less than 4.0 and which is a non-irritant to veins. Once
injected into the bloodstream, at physiological pH, it becomes
lipid soluble and is readily able to penetrate the blood-brain
barrier. It has an elimination half-life of 1.9 hours (+/−0.9 hours)
so that complete recovery is quicker than that with diazepam.
Midazolam is more rapidly acting, at least 2.5 times as potent
and has more predictable amnesic properties, than diazepam.
It is rapidly metabolised in the liver but there is also some
extra-hepatic metabolism in the bowel. Midazolam produces

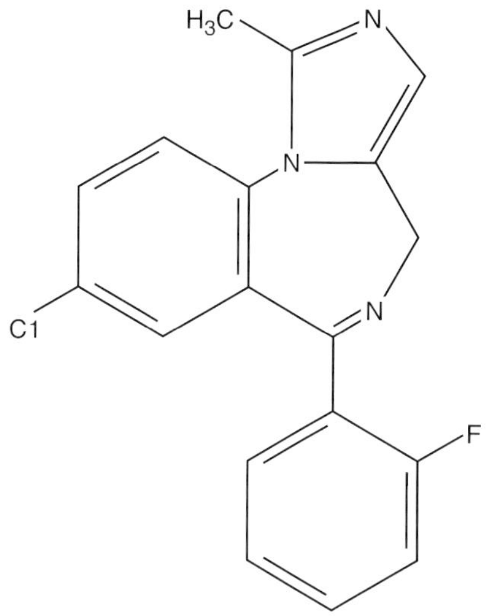

Midzolam

Figure 4.7
Chemical structure of
midazolam, showing a
benzene ring structure
attached to the diazepine
part of the molecule.

an active metabolite called alpha-hydroxymidazolam. This
has a short half-life of 1.25 hours (+/−0.25 hours) which is less
than that of the parent compound and thus does not produce
true rebound sedation. It does, however, explain the clinically
observable phenomenon of a slower initial recovery from
midazolam sedation than would be expected, on the basis of
the pharmacokinetics of the drug, without reference to its
active metabolite.

Midazolam is available in two formulations: a concentration
of 5mg/ml in a 2ml ampoule, or a concentration of 2mg/ml in
a 5ml ampoule. Both presentations contain the same quantity
of midazolam but the 5ml ampoule presentation, being less
concentrated, is easier to titrate and is more acceptable for use
in dental practice. The dose of midazolam is titrated according
to the patient's response but most patients require a dose
usually in the range of 0.07−0.1mg/kg.

Flumazenil (benzodiazepine antagonist)

The discovery of the benzodiazepine antagonist, flumazenil,
in 1978, was a major advance in the practice of intravenous
sedation. It was the first drug to effectively and completely
reverse the effects of almost all benzodiazepines. Flumazenil
is a true benzodiazepine but it has virtually no intrinsic
therapeutic activity (the administration of huge doses of
flumazenil may result in very slight epileptiform activity). It
shares the same basic chemical form as other benzodiazepines
but it lacks the ring structure attached to the diazepine part of
the molecule (Figure 4.8).

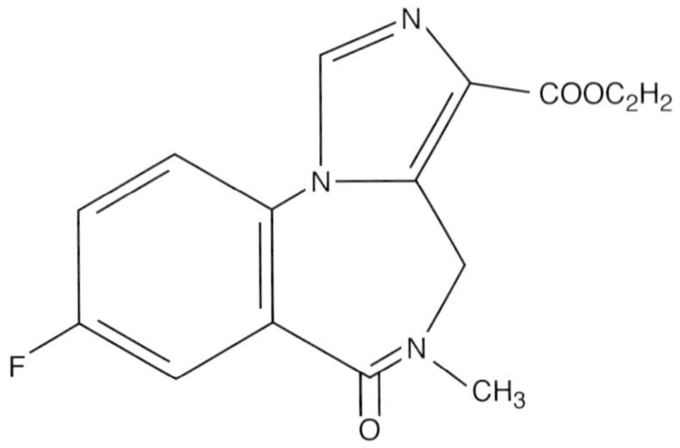

Figure 4.8
Chemical structure
of flumazenil, the
benzodiazepine
antagonist. The molecule
has no benzene ring
attached to the diazepine
group.

Flumazenil

It is this slight alteration in structure which prevents flumazenil from having any genuine therapeutic activity. Flumazenil has a greater affinity for the benzodiazepine receptor than virtually all the known active drugs and it is therefore an effective antagonist. It will reverse (at least on a temporary basis) the sedative, cardiovascular and respiratory depressant effects of both diazepam and midazolam – in fact the vast majority of all commercially available enzodiazepines.

Flumazenil is presented in 5ml ampoules containing 500mcg/ml for intravenous injection. It is administered by giving 200mcg and then waiting for 1 minute. A further 100mcg is then given every minute until the patient appears fully recovered. In an acute emergency there is no reason why higher initial doses of up to 500mcg should not be given immediately as a bolus. Flumazenil is currently only recommended for use in emergency situations and not as a means of hastening recovery. If flumazenil were used for routine reversal, there is a theoretical risk that that the benzodiazepine sedation may recur once the effect of the flumazenil had worn off. This is because flumazenil has a shorter elimination half-life (53 minutes, +/−13 minutes) than the active benzodiazepines. For healthy patients this is a theoretical concept with little basis in clinical practice and the greatest objections to using flumazenil routinely are its cost and the rather sudden and unpleasant 'wakening' which it produces. In patients who use benzodiazpines on a long-term basis, it may be significantly more problematic.

The characteristics of all three benzodiazepines considered can be seen in Table 4.1.

Other intravenous sedation agents

Although the benzodiazepines are the mainstay of modern sedation practice, they do not fulfil all the requirements of the

Table 4.1 Properties of main benzodiazepine drugs used for sedation

Benzodiazepine	Presentation	Dose Range	Metabolites	T1/2a	T1/2b
Diazepam (Diazemuls)	Emulsified, non irritant suspension in soya bean oil 2ml (5mg/ml)	0.1–0.2mg/kg	Desmethyldiazepam T1/2b (72 hrs)	40 mins	43hrs(+/–13hrs)
Midazolam	Water soluble with a pH of less than 4.0 and non-irritant 2ml (5mg/ml) 5ml (2mg/ml)	0.06–0.1 mg/kg	a-hydroxymidazolam T1/2b (1.25hrs +/–0.25)	15–30mins	1.9 hrs (+/–0.9hrs)
Flumazenil	Water soluble, non-irritant 5ml (500mcg/ml)	0.1–1mg	de-ethylated free acid and its glucuronide conjugate (inactive)	7–15 mins	53mins(+/–13 mins)

ideal sedation drug. The main problem is the relatively long period of recovery that is required before a patient can be discharged home and return to normal daily activities. To date there is only one drug which appears to have serious potential as the sedation agent of the future.

Propofol (2, 6-diisopropylphenol) is a potent intravenous hypnotic agent which is widely used for the induction and maintenance of anaesthesia and for sedation in the intensive care unit. Propofol is an oil at room temperature and insoluble in aqueous solution. Present formulations consist of 1% or 2% (w/v) propofol, 10% soya bean oil, 2.25% glycerol, and 1.2% egg phosphatide. It is presented as an aqueous white emulsion at a concentration of 10mg/ml in 20ml ampoules.

It has the advantage of undergoing rapid elimination and recovery with an elimination half-life of 30–40 minutes. It has a distribution half-life of 2–4 minutes and duration of clinical effect is short because propofol is rapidly distributed into peripheral tissues, and its effects wear off considerably within half an hour of injection. This, together with its rapid effect (within minutes of injection) and the moderate amnesia it induces, makes it an ideal drug for intravenous sedation. Propofol (Diprivan®) appears to act by enhancing the GABA neurotransmitter system.

For maintenance of general anaesthesia, propofol is administered as a continuous infusion. Following completion of the operative procedure, the infusion is stopped and the patient regains consciousness within a few minutes. Propofol may be administered in sub-anaesthetic doses either by a technique using a target-controlled infusion, a patient-controlled target infusion or by intermittent bolus administration. The propofol target-controlled infusion (TCI) system consists of an infusion pump containing software simulating the best pharmacokinetic model for propofol (Figures 4.9 and 4.10).

The patient's age and weight are programmed into the software and the desired target blood propofol concentration is selected. On commencing the infusion, a precisely calculated bolus dose is delivered to generate the selected target blood propofol concentration, followed by a continuous propofol infusion calculated to maintain that concentration. The target concentration can be increased or decreased depending on the patient's response. If a higher target concentration is selected, the pump will automatically deliver an additional bolus of propofol, followed by an increased infusion rate to maintain the increased target concentration. If a lower target concentration is selected, the pump will cease infusing propofol until it predicts that the blood propofol level has fallen to the new value, whereupon a lower infusion rate is

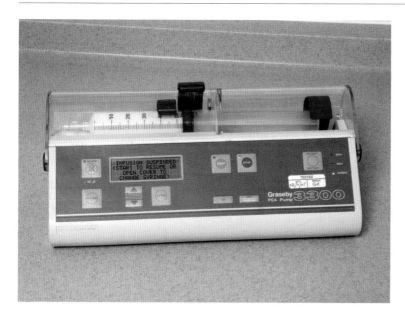

Figure 4.9
Infusion pump used for
the delivery of propofol
sedation.

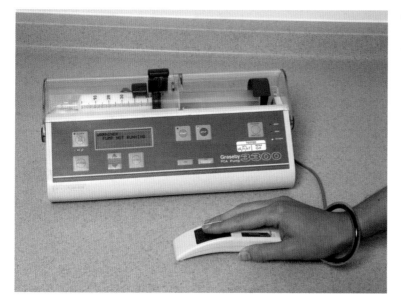

Figure 4.10
Button used by patient to
administer propofol.

delivered. Once treatment is complete, the infusion is switched
off and the patient normally will be fully recovered and fit to
be discharged home within 10–15 minutes. Target-controlled
infusion techniques have been described for sedation for a
variety of diagnostic and therapeutic procedures, including
dental surgery.

Clinical trials using propofol in differing ways for dental
sedation have been promising. Incremental doses of propofol

are administered initially until a satisfactory level of sedation is achieved, usually at a total dose of around 0.5mg/kg. The desired level of sedation is maintained by delivering a continuous infusion of around 1.5mg/kg/hr. The infusion rate can be adjusted to vary the level of sedation as required. Clinical trials using propofol, administered through a patient-controlled infusion pump (similar to those used for post-operative analgesia), have also been very promising.

In many ways, propofol approaches the requirements of an ideal sedation agent. However, it does have a number of disadvantages. The margin of safety between sedation and anaesthesia is far narrower than that of the benzodiazepines. Special equipment is also needed as the administration of propofol is by continuous infusion, requiring the use of a special infusion pump. Injection of propofol can also be painful and it should preferably be delivered into larger veins or following pre-injection with a local anaesthetic. The use of propofol for dental sedation is essentially still at the experimental stage and as such it can only be recommended for use in a hospital environment. Its continued development may see it eventually become more commonly used in sedation practice, since it has certainly gained wide acceptance in its use as an induction agent for general anaesthesia, but at the present time it cannot be recommended as a drug suitable for a safe operator-sedation technique.

References and further reading

Calvey, N. & Williams, N.E. (2008) *Principles and Practice of Pharmacology for Anaesthetists*, 5th edn. Oxford, Blackwell Scientific Publishing.

Girdler, N.M., Rynn, D., Lyne, J.P. & Wilson, K.E. (2000) A prospective randomised controlled study of patient-controlled propfol sedation in phobic dental patients. *Anaesthesia*, **55**(4), 327–33.

Goodchild, C.S. (1993) GABA receptors and benzodiazepines. *British Journal of Anaesthesia*, **71**(1), 127–133.

Leitch, J.A., Sutcliffe, N. & Kenny, G.N. (2003) Patient-maintained sedation for oral surgery using a target-controlled infusion of propofol – a pilot study. *British Dental Journal*, **194**(1), 43–5.

Maze, M. & Fujinaga, M. (2000) Recent advances in understanding the actions and toxicity of nitrous oxide. *Anaesthesia*, **55**, 311–314.

Yagiela, J.A. (1991) Health hazards and nitrous oxide: a time for reappraisal. *Anaesthesia Progress*, **38**, 1–11.

5 Premedication and oral sedation

PREMEDICATION

Premedication refers to a drug treatment given to a patient prior to a surgical or invasive medical procedure, to obtain anxiolysis. These drugs are typically sedatives. However, premedications can also be used on occasion for other reasons, such as reducing salivary and bronchial secretions, lessening the response to painful stimuli and reducing the risk of vomiting, particularly prior to general anaesthesia.

When considering the management of anxious patients under conscious sedation, premedication is used for producing pre-operative anxiolysis and is generally given by the oral route. Such premedication may be indicated in the following cases:

- To reduce anxiety the night before the appointment
- To reduce anxiety in the 1–2 hours period before treatment
- For patients who are needle phobic, but require intravenous sedation for treatment.

Drugs used for pre-operative anxiolysis

Several agents can be used for premedication but the benzodiazepines are the most commonly used.

Diazepam

Until recently, diazepam was the most commonly and widely used of all sedatives for premedication. It is available in tablets of 2mg, 5mg and 10mg and is fairly reliably absorbed from the gut, its effects becoming apparent after about 30 minutes. The correct dosage for each individual is not easy to calculate, since several factors influence its action. In particular, it does appear to bear a relationship to the age of a patient, much higher (relative) dosages being required in children and adolescents. As with intravenous administration, the converse is true in the elderly and infirm. As a rough guide, a dose between 0.1mg and 0.25mg/kg of body weight will produce adequate anxiolysis and should be given 1 hour before surgery and after a light snack. Administration of a single dose of oral diazepam, does give the operator the opportunity to form a baseline assessment, on which further action may be taken. Too high a dosage will cause sleep, whilst inadequate dosage will result in an alert and still anxious patient. Potential side effects include dizziness, increased pain awareness, ataxia (difficulty maintaining posture) and occasional respiratory depression. Prolonged post-operative drowsiness has also been reported.

Caution is necessary in administering diazepam to patients with obvious psychoses, neuromuscular disorders, or respiratory, liver or kidney disease. Alcohol intake must be prohibited for a period of 24 hours before and after administration. Patients should not drive or operate machinery for 24 hours post-medication. As with intravenous diazepam, there is also some risk of some re-sedation after 2–3 days due to the production of active metabolites. Oral diazepam has been found particularly useful in the treatment of patients with cerebral palsy, coupling it with intravenous midazolam as the main sedation agent.

Temazepam

Temazepam is now one of the most commonly used oral premedication agents. It was originally marketed as a hypnotic for inducing sleep but its shorter half-life (circa 4 hours) makes it ideal for use as an anxyolitic. An anxious, otherwise healthy adult of normal weight should be given a dose of 10mg and the effect assessed after 30 minutes. The dose may be doubled for severely anxious patients.

ORAL SEDATION

Oral sedation, in contrast to oral premedication, is a technique where an oral drug is administered to produce a state of conscious sedation, where the patient will allow treatment to be carried out and differs from premedication, which is designed to produce mild anxiolysis only. Oral sedation offers a non-threatening approach to sedation as it does not require an injection to administer. It may be considered more versatile than inhalation sedation, since it does not require the same amount of patient co-operation in the initial stages.

The ideal oral sedative would clearly fit the general criteria for sedation and would, therefore:

1. Alleviate fear and anxiety
2. Not suppress protective reflexes
3. Be easy to administer
4. Be quickly effective
5. Be free of side effects
6. Be predictable in duration and action
7. Be quickly metabolised and excreted
8. Not produce active metabolites
9. Have an active half-life of approximately 45–60 minutes.

It is difficult to find any drug that fits all the above criteria, and some of the features mentioned above are much easier to control in inhalation and intravenous sedation than they are with oral sedation. This is because of the variation in predictability that inevitably occurs in relation to:
1. An individual's degree of anxiety
2. The pattern of absorption of the drug
3. The rate of metabolism of the drug.

This leads to considerable individual variation in response, which means that the outcome of many oral sedatives is less predictable than agents (even of the same chemical formulation) which are given parenterally. Oral sedation should only be considered where intravenous or inhalation sedation are not appropriate or have been unsuccessful.

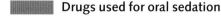 ## Drugs used for oral sedation

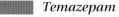 ### *Temazepam*

As well as its use as a premedication agent, temazepam can be used to produce oral sedation in adults when used in higher doses such as 30–40 mg. When used in this way, the patient's vital signs must be monitored throughout the period of sedation and treatment.

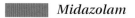 ### *Midazolam*

Midazolam is a potentially useful drug for providing oral sedation for the dental patient, however it is not licensed for this route of administration and its use must be fully justified following consideration of other management options. It is available in the oral form as an elixir in certain countries. The injectable form can be prepared by local hospital pharmacy units for use orally. It can also be mixed with fruit cordial or syrup to make it more palatable for providing oral sedation.

Taken orally, midazolam has an onset time of approximately 20–30 minutes. Some of the drug will be absorbed in the gastrointestinal tract and liver ('first pass metabolism') and as a result of this only a proportion of the drug reaches the circulation. The effects will therefore vary on an individual basis depending on the degree of first pass metabolism which takes place. Similarly, recovery times are variable and it is essential to keep the patient in recovery until they fully meet the desired discharge criteria. It is advisable when using oral midazolam to place an intravenous cannula so that, in the case of an emergency, flumazenil or other emergency drugs can be easily administered.

SUMMARY

The techniques of oral premedication and oral sedation have been presented. It should be emphasised that they are two separate therapeutic techniques and require appropriate knowledge and training to be competent in their use.

6 Principles and practice of inhalation sedation

Inhalation sedation is the safest form of sedation, due principally to the nature of nitrous oxide, which is almost universally used in this technique. The term 'inhalation sedation' describes the induction of a state of conscious sedation by administering sub-anaesthetic concentrations of gaseous anaesthetic agents. Its most common application is in children's dentistry, where it has been used successfully for many decades, but its use in adult dentistry is increasing. The favourable pharmacological properties of nitrous oxide make it the agent of choice for most inhalation sedation techniques.

Since its discovery in the eighteenth century, nitrous oxide has been the basic constituent of gaseous general anaesthesia, although it was not until the 1960s that it was more widely used in inhalation sedation. Harold Langa of the United States introduced the concept of 'relative analgesia', a specific type of inhalation sedation. This sedation uses variable mixtures of nitrous oxide and oxygen to induce a state of psycho-pharmacological sedation that was previously classified as stage 1 of anaesthesia. The staging of anaesthesia was described in 1937 when Arthur Guedel detailed the physical level, or depth, of patients' anaesthesia with ether. Langa later developed the concept of planes of sedation within stage 1 of anaesthesia. Though the stages are still found in most standard anaesthesia textbooks, they are unrecognisable from Guedel's, with the use of modern, rapidly effective agents.

Relative analgesia has now become the standard technique for inhalation sedation in dentistry. Other methods of inhalation sedation do exist, such as the use of fixed concentrations of nitrous oxide and oxygen (Entonox®) but these are not commonly used in dentistry.

▨▨▨▨ INHALATION SEDATION IN DENTISTRY

The aims of inhalation sedation are to alleviate fear by producing anxiolysis, to reduce pain by inducing analgesia, and to improve patient co-operation so that dental treatment can be performed. Inhalation sedation embodies a triad of elements:

1. The administration of low to moderate titrated concentrations of nitrous oxide in oxygen to patients who remain conscious
2. The use of a specifically designed machine with a number of safety features, including the ability to deliver a minimum of 30% oxygen and a fail-safe device that cuts off the delivery of nitrous oxide if the oxygen supply fails
3. The use of semi-hypnotic suggestion to reassure and encourage the patient throughout the period of sedation and treatment.

The success of inhalation sedation relies on a balanced combination of pharmacology and behaviour management. Nitrous oxide (N_2O) will produce a degree of pharmacological sedation on its own but this is unpredictable and should be supplemented and reinforced with psychological reassurance. The pharmacological properties of nitrous oxide produce physiological changes which enhance the patient's susceptibility to suggestion. The use of semi-hypnotic suggestion to positively reinforce feelings of relaxation and well-being, will increase the extent of the anxiolysis and co-operation. In contrast to intravenous sedation, which produces pharmacological sedation regardless of any element of suggestion, inhalation sedation induces a state of psycho-pharmacological sedation.

▨▨▨▨ Planes of analgesia

The clinical effects of sedation with nitrous oxide can be divided into three broad categories. These form part of the stages of anaesthesia (Figure 6.1).

The first stage of anaesthesia, the analgesic stage, is subdivided into three 'planes of analgesia':

Plane I   Moderate sedation and analgesia, obtained at concentrations of 5–25% nitrous oxide.

Plane II   Dissociation sedation and analgesia, occurring at concentrations of 20–55% nitrous oxide.

Plane III   Total analgesia, obtained with concentrations of nitrous oxide usually well above 50%.

In general terms, most clinically useful sedation is produced in Plane I and sometimes in Plane II, although some patients find the dissociation effects disorientating. It is these planes that are

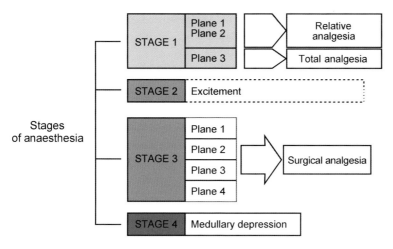

Figure 6.1
Guedel's stages of anaesthesia. Stage 1 is subdivided into three planes of analgesia.

encompassed by the definition of relative analgesia (inhalation sedation). Plane III is a transition zone between the state of conscious sedation and true general anaesthesia and thus it is termed total analgesia rather than relative analgesia. There is considerable overlap between the planes and a large variation in susceptibility of individual patients to the effects of nitrous oxide. Whilst one person may be adequately sedated with 10% nitrous oxide, another individual may require in excess of 50% nitrous oxide to achieve the same degree of sedation.

Each plane of analgesia is accompanied by specific clinical signs:

Plane I (N_2O concentrations of 5–25%)

- relaxation and a general sense of well-being
- paraesthesia, a tingling feeling in the fingers, toes and cheeks
- a feeling of suffusing warmth is common
- alert and readily responds to questioning
- slight reduction in spontaneous movements
- decreased reaction to painful stimuli
- pulse, blood pressure, respiration rate, reflexes and pupil reactions will all be normal.

As the nitrous oxide concentration is increased to the 20–55% range there will be a gradual transition from Plane I to Plane II.

Plane II (N_2O concentrations of 20–55%)

- marked relaxation and sleepiness
- a feeling of detachment from the environment
- senses will be altered
- possible dreaming

- widespread paraesthesia, moderate analgesia
- reduction in the gag reflex
- delayed response to questioning
- vital signs and the laryngeal reflexes should be unaffected.

When the nitrous oxide concentration goes above 50%, there will normally be a transition into Plane III.

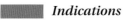 Plane III (N_2O concentrations above 50%)

- marked sleepiness and a 'glazed' appearance
- complete analgesia
- nausea and dizziness are common
- patient may vomit
- unresponsive to questioning
- may lose consciousness and enter Stage 2 of general anaesthesia.

If any of these signs occur, the nitrous oxide level should be reduced. There is usually a gradual transition between planes and not all patients show all of the clinical signs. However, the planes of analgesia are a useful guide to what to expect when sedating a patient with nitrous oxide. Specific signs such as nausea, dizziness and a glazed appearance provide a warning that the level of sedation is too high and the percentage of nitrous oxide should be reduced. However, there is considerable variation in individual response and it should be remembered that the success of the technique is probably more dependent on the operator's ability to infuse hypnotic suggestion, than it is to the effect of nitrous oxide.

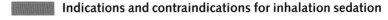 Indications and contraindications for inhalation sedation

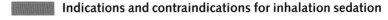 Indications

- Management of dental anxiety (children and adults)
- Management of needle phobia
- Management of gag reflex
- Management of medically compromised patients.

Inhalation sedation is particularly useful for anxious children. Children must be able to understand the purpose and mechanisms (in appropriate terminology) of inhalation sedation, so the minimum age for treating children under inhalation sedation is approximately three years. This is usually the lowest age at which the child has an appropriate degree of understanding to enable sufficient co-operation for treatment.

Older children scheduled for orthodontic extractions may also benefit from inhalation sedation. Such children may not be particularly frightened of routine treatment but multiple extractions of permanent teeth or surgical procedures, such as the exposure of canines, can be somewhat traumatic. Sedation can help to make the procedure more acceptable and the time pass more quickly.

Another key indication for inhalation sedation is the treatment of adults who have a general (as opposed to dental) phobia of needles or injections. Such individuals find it impossible to accept venepuncture and venous cannulation. They can benefit considerably from inhalation sedation, either as the sole form of sedation or in combination with intravenous sedation. In many cases, the level of sedation and analgesia achieved with inhalation sedation is sufficient for the patient to receive a local anaesthetic injection into the mucosa with minimal discomfort and simple operative dentistry can then be performed. However, for patients with a severe anxiety or phobia of dentistry, it may be necessary to supplement inhalation sedation with an intravenous technique. In these individuals the inhalation sedation is used to induce a level of sedation sufficient to enable venous cannulation. Once the cannula is successfully located, the intravenous sedative can be administered and the delivery of nitrous oxide terminated.

Inhalation sedation is also used for a number of special categories of patients who are at risk from the respiratory depressive effects of intravenous agents. These include patients with sickle cell anaemia or asthma, who benefit from the guaranteed level of oxygenation (at least 30% and usually significantly more) used in inhalation sedation. For the few patients with a proven allergy to intravenous sedatives, the only alternative sedation technique may be inhalation sedation.

Contraindications

Many of the contraindications to inhalation sedation are relative or temporary and include:
* upper respiratory tract infections
* large tonsils or adenoids
* serious respiratory disease
* mouth breathers
* very young children
* moderate to severe learning difficulties
* severe psychiatric disorders
* pregnant women
* upper anterior apicectomy.

Very few of the indications and contraindications for inhalation sedation are absolute. In many cases it is necessary to carefully balance the risk of giving the patient sedation against the risk of general anaesthesia, which is often the only option for many anxious dental patients. Each patient should be individually assessed, although only those who fit the above selection criteria and who meet the general standards discussed in Chapter 3, should be treated in dental practice. There may be others, however, who can be referred for treatment under inhalation sedation in a hospital setting, where any complications can be dealt with more easily.

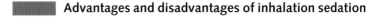 **Advantages and disadvantages of inhalation sedation**

Advantages

- Non-invasive technique with no requirement for venepuncture/ cannulation
- Nitrous oxide is relatively inert so that there are no metabolic demands
- The low solubility of nitrous oxide ensures a rapid onset and recovery
- The level of sedation can easily be altered or discontinued
- Little effect on the cardiovascular and respiratory systems
- Some analgesia produced.

Disadvantages

- The drug is administered continuously via a nose mask close to the operative site
- The mask may be objectionable to the patient
- The level of sedation relies heavily on psychological reassurance
- The technique requires a certain level of compliance in terms of breathing through the nose
- It is not suitable for very young children and patients with learning difficulties.

Patient preparation for inhalation sedation

Assessment and treatment planning for patients for inhalation sedation should follow the format described earlier in Chapter 3. The main difference is that most patients presenting for inhalation sedation are children. Inhalation sedation should be seen as part of an overall behaviour management strategy and the aim of the assessment appointment should be to select those patients who need some form of extra support to help them through treatment. When assessing children for inhalation sedation it is important to involve both the child and the parent.

The type and extent of dental treatment needed should be taken into account when considering sedation. Although most routine operative dentistry can be performed under inhalation sedation, the nature of the treatment must be matched against the age of the patient and their predicted level of co-operation. One or two extractions in a four-year-old could, quite reasonably, be performed under inhalation sedation. However, if the same patient required the extraction of multiple grossly carious teeth it might be kinder to refer the patient for a short general anaesthetic. Similarly, a 13-year-old could willingly accept the extraction of four premolars under inhalation sedation, but if they required the exposure of a deeply buried canine, general anaesthesia may be preferable.

Assessment of the medical status of a patient scheduled for inhalation sedation is identical to that described in Chapter 3. Particular attention should be paid to respiratory disease, as this can affect ventilation and gas exchange. The patient should be examined to check patency of the nasal air passages. A baseline pulse and respiration rate should be recorded but, for healthy patients, it is unnecessary to take the weight and blood pressure.

Pre-operative instructions

A full explanation of the procedure should be given to the patient–and the parent where the patient is a child. For children it is important to explain the procedure using simple terminology. Children should be told that they will be given some 'happy air' or 'magic wind' to breath, which will make them feel 'warm', 'tingly' and 'sleepy'. Once they feel comfortable then their tooth will be 'washed' to make it 'tingly'. It will then be 'wiggled out' or 'mended'. The truth should always be told, although the use of careful semantics is extremely important. Children should be reassured that they will be able to talk to the dentist while they are sedated. Clearly the level of explanation should be individually pitched according to the age and level of understanding of the child. The parent, guardian or patient (if over the age of 16 years) should be asked to sign a written consent to both the sedation and dental treatment.

Full spoken and written instructions about pre- and post-operative care should be given to the parent or to the patient (if over 16 years old) including the need for
- A light meal 2 hours before the appointment
- Children to be accompanied by a responsible adult
- Transport home in car or taxi

- Children should not ride bikes, drive vehicles or operate machinery for the rest of the day
- Children should be supervised by an adult for the rest of the day.

Adults who are undergoing inhalation sedation, as the sole method of sedation, do not need to be accompanied. Once they are deemed fit for discharge, adults can go home alone, although it is inadvisable for them to drive.

Equipment for inhalation sedation

Machines have been designed specifically for providing inhalation sedation in the dental surgery. They may be either free-standing units or piped gas units. Various makes are available in the UK including the Quantiflex MDM®, Digital MDM Mixer® (Electronic), and Porter MXR Flowmeters. They allow a variable percentage of nitrous oxide and oxygen to be delivered to the patient via a nose mask. The gas flow is continuous but the rate can be individually adjusted to match the patient's minute volume.

Free-standing units

Free-standing units carry their own gas supply: two cylinders of nitrous oxide and two cylinders of oxygen (Figure 6.2). One cylinder of each gas is in active use and the second cylinder is a reserve supply which must always be kept full and should be labelled accordingly. The cylinders are attached to the machine with a specific pin-index connection which prevents attachment of the wrong gas cylinders. Gas leaving the cylinders goes through a pressure-reducing valve before passing into a flow control head.

Piped gas unit

Piped units consist of a pipeline system which supplies the nitrous oxide and oxygen from remote cylinders held in appropriate storage units (Figure 6.3).

Sedation unit head

Both free-standing and piped systems house the same head units, depending on the manufacturer (Figure 6.4).

The flow rate of each gas can be visualised in two flow meters on the control head, each calibrated in one litre increments up to 10 litres per minute. The nitrous oxide and oxygen are mixed in the flow control head. A flow control knob regulates the rate at which the gas mixture is delivered to the patient, and mixture

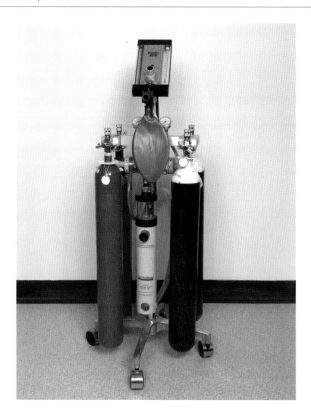

Figure 6.2
Free-standing inhalation
sedation machine.

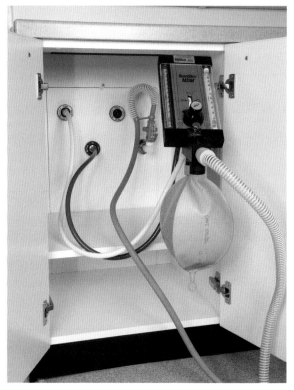

Figure 6.3
Piped inhalation sedation
system.

Figure 6.4
Quantiflex MDM®, flow control head, showing nitrous oxide and oxygen flow meters, mixture control dial, flow control knob and oxygen flush button.

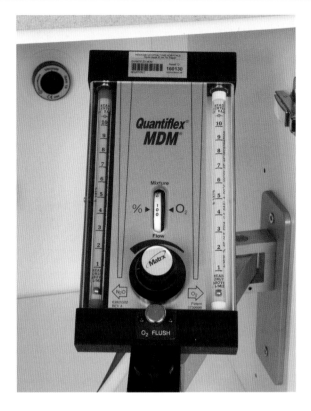

control dials determine the relative percentage of nitrous oxide and oxygen being delivered to the patient. On the Quantiflex MDM head the mixture control dial actually indicates the percentage of oxygen being administered and is marked in 10% increments, from 100% down to 30% (the minimum level). As the oxygen concentration is changed, the balance of the gas mixture is automatically made to 100% with nitrous oxide. On the Porter system there are separate control dials for nitrous oxide and oxygen. The control head also contains an air entrainment valve which opens automatically to let air in if there is any negative pressure in the breathing circuit. So if the gas flow rate is inadvertently set too low for a particular patient, the air entrainment valve will open, so that the patient can breathe room air in addition to the delivered gas volume.

Reservoir bag

After leaving the flow control head the gas mixture enters a reservoir bag, which should be latex free (Figure 6.5). The reservoir bag has three main purposes:
- It allows the flow rate to be accurately adjusted to match the patient's minute volume. If the bag empties whilst the

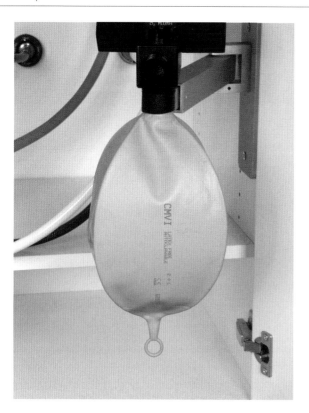

Figure 6.5
The reservoir bag is situated just below the flow control head.

patient breathes, then the flow rate is set too low for that patient's minute volume. In contrast, if the bag is continuously over-inflated, then the flow rate is set too high. Ideally the reservoir bag should stay about three-quarters full, deflating slightly as the patient inspires and refilling as the patient expires.

- As an adjunct to clinical monitoring. Regular observation of movement of the bag during treatment allows the respiration rate and depth to be monitored.
- For manual positive pressure ventilation in the event of an emergency. This can only be effective if the valves on the mask and in the breathing system are first closed.

Gas delivery system

The gas mixture is administered to the patient via a gas delivery hose attached to the input port of a suitable nasal mask. There are various sizes of rubber nose masks available and it is important to select one which provides the best seal with the patient's face (Figure 6.6).

A poorly fitting mask will allow gas to escape, which decreases the efficiency of the sedation and leads to pollution

Figure 6.6
Inhalation sedation nose mask, showing the inner and outer units.

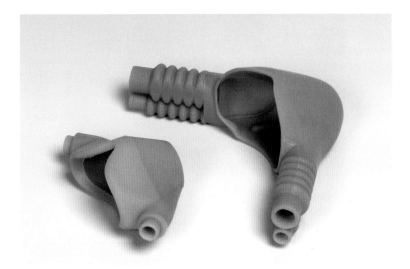

of the dental surgery. The patient inhales fresh gas from the mask and then exhales waste gas back into the mask. Exhaled gas passes through the output port in the mask to a scavenging hose. A one-way valve in the scavenging hose or mask system prevents waste gas from being re-inhaled. The exhaled gas is actively removed by a customised scavenging system.

Safety features of inhalation sedation equipment:

1. **Minimum oxygen delivery:** The machine is constructed so that the minimum oxygen delivery is 30% of total gas volume, regardless of the total volume of gases flowing. This will ensure the patient always receives a gas mixture with a higher percentage of oxygen than is present in normal room air (>21%), virtually eliminating the risk of inducing full anaesthesia.
2. **Automatic gas cut-out:** An automatic cut-out of all gas delivery occurs if the oxygen supply fails or if the oxygen delivery falls below 30%. This would only occur if the oxygen cylinder ran out of gas or if there was blockage or leakage in the high pressure system. This feature also ensures that 100% nitrous oxide can never be delivered to the patient.
3. **Colour coding:** All components associated with nitrous oxide are coloured blue, and oxygen white. This includes the flow-meter gauge, the tubing from the cylinder and/or the gas outlet to the pressure-reducing valve.
4. **Pin index system:** On the free-standing unit this system ensures that oxygen and nitrous oxide cylinders cannot be interchanged. On the piped unit the sizes of the oxygen and nitrous oxide wall outlets differ.
5. **Gas pressure dials:** The pressure dials enable the operator to ensure sufficient gas supplies are available before and during treatment.

6. **Audible alarm:** An alarm should be audible to indicate when oxygen levels are falling.
7. **Scavenging:** Active scavenging units must be available to reduce pollution of the surgery with nitrous oxide.

Equipment checks

The inhalation sedation machine and associated apparatus should always be thoroughly checked before use:

Gas levels: For the free-standing unit, each oxygen cylinder must be separately switched on and the pressure dial checked. One cylinder at least should be completely full and any cylinders showing low readings should be changed. The flow rate should be turned on to maximum and the dial re-checked to ensure that there is no decrease in pressure. If such a decrease occurs, it would indicate that either the quantity of gas in the cylinder is low or there is an obstruction in the high pressure part of the system. The full cylinder should then be switched off and labelled as full. Cylinders of nitrous oxide need to be weighed to confirm the quantity of gas. Nitrous oxide is stored as a liquid under pressure and the pressure dial will not accurately indicate the amount of liquid in the cylinder. The ability of the cylinders to deliver a sufficient flow of gas should also be tested. It is more practical when the unit is first set up to ensure the full and in-use labels are appropriately placed and these are always checked when cylinders are replaced.

Leaks in system: A check should be made for leaks in the system by occluding the nose mask with one hand, allowing the reservoir bag to fill up and then squeezing it hard. The bag should not deflate unless gas is forced through the nose mask past the occluding hand. Any other deflation of the bag indicates a leakage.

Automatic gas cut-out: For the free-standing unit the effectiveness of the safety cut-out should be tested by switching on both the oxygen and nitrous oxide, setting the mixture control dial to 50% oxygen/50% nitrous oxide and the flow rate to 8 litres/minute. When the oxygen cylinder is turned off, the nitrous oxide should automatically cut-out within a few seconds. For the piped system, to cut off the oxygen supply, the wall outlet supply should be disconnected.

Oxygen flush button: The oxygen flush button should be tested to ensure a flow of gas is produced when it is activated.

Gas tubing and one-way valves: The gas tubing should be inspected for tears or perishing and the one-way valve in the expiratory limb or mask of the breathing system should be in place.

Gas supply activated: For the free-standing unit the correct cylinders should be switched on and their valves opened fully.

For the piped system ensure the gas hosing is connected to the wall outlets.

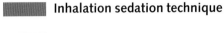 **Inhalation sedation technique**

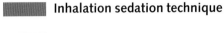 *Pre-operative checks*

Before escorting the patient to the surgery, a checklist (Figure 6.7) should be completed and signed and should include:
- Patient's name and date of birth
- Date of procedure
- Operating dentist and assisting dental nurse
- Equipment present and checked including
  - Dental equipment
  - Sedation equipment
  - Emergency equipment
- Patient checks
  - Patient knows what is planned
  - Consent obtained
  - Medical history up to date
  - Patient has not fasted for longer than 2 hours
  - No alcohol has been consumed in the previous 24 hours
  - Escort available
  - Transport home available.

 Patient management

The patient should then be brought into the surgery by the dental nurse and settled in the dental chair. The procedure for inhalation sedation is explained and the patient is shown the nasal mask (Figure 6.8).

The patient is encouraged to try it on so that an appropriate size can be selected. It is important to tell the patient about the positive feelings they will have during sedation. They should be reassured that they will be able to talk to the dentist during treatment.

It is better to recline the patient into a supine position before starting the sedation, as this makes the technique easier and minimises the risk of fainting. Once the patient is comfortable, 100% oxygen is allowed to flow through the system at approximately 4 litres/minute for children and 6 litres/minute for adults. The patient is then asked to place the nose mask to allow the patient to feel in control and part of the process. The clinician then ensures the mask fits well to avoid gas leaks (Figure 6.9).

The patient is asked to try and keep his/her mouth closed and to breathe slowly and regularly. Constant reassurance should be given. By observing the movement of the reservoir

INHALATIONAL SEDATION TREATMENT RECORD	Affix patient identification label in box below or complete details	
	Surname	Patient ID No.
	Forename	D.O.B. D D M M Y Y Y Y
	Address	NHS No.
		Sex. Male / Female
	Postcode	

Date	
Clinician - Sedationist - Operator	
Assistant(s)	

PRE-SEDATION CHECKLIST

1. Staff Check:	
Experienced qualified assistant present?	
Clinician/assistant know emergency procedure?	
2. Emergency and Monitoring Equipment Check:	
Site of Emergency Equipment known	
Oxygen - emergency/routine	
Suction - fixed/mobile - back up	
Positive pressure ventilating bag	
Pulse oximeter and Sphygmomanometer	
ECG/defibrillator	
Emergency drugs	
3. Relative Analgesia Equipment Check:	
Oxygen and nitrous oxide cylinders	
Pressure gauges, flowmeters	
Automatic nitrous oxide cut-out	
Reservoir bag, gas tubing, nose mask	
Scavenging equipment	
4. Patient Check:	
Patient and parent understand what is planned	
Written consent obtained	
Medical history check	
Normal medication taken	
Last meal/drink	
Escort and transport	

Figure 6.7 Pre-procedural checklist for inhalation sedation.

Figure 6.8
The nose mask is shown
to the patient and the
procedure explained.

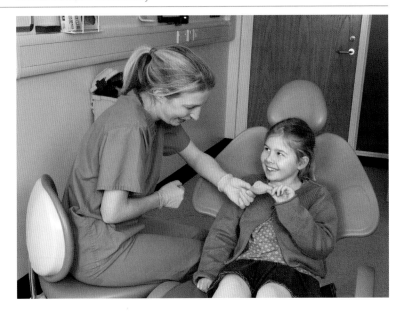

Figure 6.9
The nose mask is
comfortably positioned
on the patient's nose. It
is important to check for
a good seal around the
mask to prevent leakage.

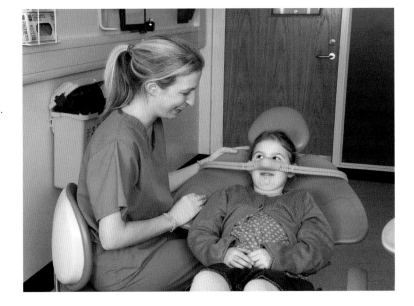

bag and asking patients if they feel comfortable, the flow rate
should be adjusted until a comfortable minute volume is
achieved.

The administration of nitrous oxide can then be slowly
introduced. Ten percent nitrous oxide is added by turning the
mixture control dial to 90% oxygen. Patients should be told that
dizziness or feeling lightheaded is normal, as is a warm tingling
in the feet and hands. They may also start to feel a little

detached from their surroundings and experience changes
in hearing and vision. At this stage it is extremely important
to reassure patients by continuous conversation and
encouragement, stressing that the feelings will be positive and
pleasant. The flow is maintained for one full minute and then
the concentration of nitrous oxide is increased by a further 10%,
to 20% (80% oxygen) for a full minute. Thereafter the level of
nitrous oxide can be increased in 5% or 10% increments to 30%
(70% oxygen), the dose being carefully titrated according to the
patient's response. If further sedation is required, it is essential
that the nitrous oxide is increased by 5% increments until the
end point is reached.

   Throughout the titration period it is mandatory to use
hypnotic suggestion in the form of story telling or positive
affirmation to distract and relax the patient. The operator
should speak in low volumes with a monotone voice.

   An adequate level of sedation is achieved when there is
general relaxation, the patient is less fidgety and less talkative,
there is tingling or paraesthesia of the fingers, toes and possibly
the lips and a slowed response to questioning is noted. When
these signs are evident the patient should be asked if they
would be happy to start treatment. A positive response is a good
indication that the end point has been achieved. The average
concentration of nitrous oxide that is used has been reported
at 30%, however concentrations between 20% and 40%,
commonly allow for a state of detached sedation and analgesia
without any loss of consciousness or danger of obtunded
laryngeal reflexes.

   If after a period of relaxation patients become restless
and apprehensive, or if they start to complain of nausea or
dizziness, this is usually an indication that the level of nitrous
oxide is too high and the patient is becoming over-sedated.
The percentage of nitrous oxide should be reduced in 5%
stages, the patient reassured and a more appropriate
level of sedation maintained until the operative procedure
is complete. If at any time the patient becomes glazed and
unresponsive to questioning, he or she is probably entering
the early stages of anaesthesia and the immediate response
should be to reduce the nitrous oxide level and provide
100% oxygen.

   Once an appropriate level of sedation has been achieved
local anaesthesia can be administered. The analgesic effect
of nitrous oxide can make local anaesthetic injections less
uncomfortable, but it is still good practice to also use a topical
anaesthetic. Administration of nitrous oxide and oxygen should
continue throughout the operative period and treatment should
be accompanied by ongoing reassurance and encouragement.
The degree of sedation may fall slightly during treatment as

there may be a degree of mouth breathing, effectively diluting the gas mixture. This can be rectified by encouraging the patient to breathe through his/her nose or by ceasing dental treatment temporarily and asking the patient to close the mouth and breathe nasally for a few minutes. On no account should a dental prop ever be used to keep the patient's mouth open during routine treatment. If a patient cannot maintain an open mouth, it is a sign that they are too deeply sedated.

Monitoring

It is essential to monitor the clinical status of the patient throughout the period of nitrous oxide sedation. Clinical monitoring of respiration rate and depth, pulse, colour, level of sedation and responsiveness are mandatory. However, in a healthy patient, it is not necessary to supplement clinical observation with electro-mechanical monitoring. Pulse oximetry and blood pressure measurement during relative analgesia are only indicated in the care of medically compromised patients, especially those with cardiac insufficiency. It is useful to have them available, however, in case of complications.

Recovery

When dental treatment is complete, the nitrous oxide flow is stopped and 100% oxygen is administered for approximately two to three minutes until the patient feels that the sedation has worn off. The aim of this is primarily to prevent 'diffusion hypoxia', a condition which results from the rapid outflow of nitrous oxide across the alveolar membrane when the incoming gas flow is stopped. This can dilute the percentage of alveolar oxygen available for uptake by up to 50%, although the risk of severe, life-threatening diffusion hypoxia is very low. The administration of 100% oxygen counteracts the potential desaturation caused by diffusion hypoxia. Finally, the patient is asked to remove the face-mask and is slowly brought back to the upright position.

Discharge

After a period of about 10–15 minutes the patient is usually fit to be discharged. The dental clinician should check that the patient is coherent, standing steady and can walk unaided. Children should be discharged into the care of an adult, with written post-operative instructions (see Figure 6.10). Adult patients can be allowed home unaccompanied once the dental clinician has confirmed their fitness to be discharged.

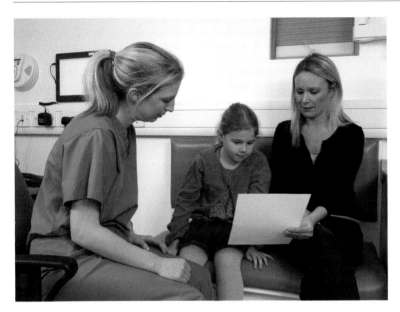

Figure 6.10
Spoken and written post-operative instructions are given to the patient and their escort.

Sedation records

The inhalation sedation procedure carried out must be fully documented in the patient's records and should include details of the percentage of oxygen and nitrous oxide delivered, the flow rate of the gases, the level of patient co-operation and the fact that 100% oxygen was administered prior to discharge. A record sheet detailing the required information is illustrated in Figure 6.11.

Safety and complications of inhalation sedation

Inhalation sedation with nitrous oxide and oxygen has an excellent safety record. To date there have been no recorded cases of significant morbidity or mortality occurring from this form of sedation in the United Kingdom. Provided that the dental clinician and assisting dental nurse are adequately trained, patients are carefully selected and the correct equipment with specific safety features is used, then inhalation sedation is a very safe and effective technique.

The principal complications associated with inhalation sedation can be divided into acute and chronic effects.

Acute effects

Acute effects are associated with the patient and include:
• Over-sedation
• Diffusion hypoxia

PROCEDURAL RECORD

Drug Administration	
Nitrous Oxide (%)	
Oxygen (%)	
Total Gas Flow Rate (litres/min)	

Monitoring Record			
Clinical Monitoring	Pre-sedation	During sedation	Recovery/ Prior to discharge
Respiration rate			
Pulse			
Level of Responsiveness			
Electro-mechanical Monitoring (if used)			
Oxygen saturation			
Blood Pressure			

Operative Details			
Co-operation			
Dental Treatment undertaken			
Complications (sedation or preoperative)			

Recovery and Discharge	
Assessment of fitness for discharge	
Written post-sedation instructions to parent/patient	
Clinician's approval to discharge	
Names of discharging - clinician - nurse	
Time of discharge	

Signature of clinician	

Figure 6.11 Treatment record sheet for inhalation sedation.

- Undue hypersensitivity to nitrous oxide
- Medical emergencies (see Chapter 8).

Chronic effects

Chronic effects are associated with chronic exposure of dental personnel to nitrous oxide and have been considered in Chapter 4. Available data do not support the notion that exposure to trace amounts of nitrous oxide is associated with biochemical changes. Although no cause and effect relationship has been firmly established, exposure to the gas should be minimised.

Reducing nitrous oxide pollution: To keep nitrous oxide pollution to a minimum in the dental surgery there are a number of recommendations to follow:

- Active scavenging – Active gas scavenging is a statutory requirement during the provision of inhalation sedation with nitrous oxide in the UK. The recognised definition of an active dental scavenging breathing system is an air flow rate of 45 litres/min at the nasal hood, which allows the removal of waste gas by the application of low power suction to the expiratory limb of the breathing circuit.
- Passive scavenging – Further ways to reduce trace levels of nitrous oxide include opening a window or door and using floor-level active fan ventilation to the exterior of the building.
- Appropriate technique – Appropriate patient selection, good seal of nasal mask, minimise patient talking during treatment.

There is a legal requirement for dental surgeons to comply with health and safety regulations. All steps should be taken to minimise unnecessary staff exposure to nitrous oxide. Pregnant women and those trying to conceive should not be allowed to work in a surgery where nitrous oxide is being used. It is imperative that a clinic protocol is written and adhered to concerning the issue of safe usage on nitrous oxide/oxygen inhalation sedation.

Despite all the precautions required and the skill needed in using inhalation sedation, it is a technique which is tried and tested and one which most patients find helpful in managing mild anxiety. Its use is likely to remain more popular in children but, as with oral sedatives, relative analgesia offers most patients a non-threatening approach to sedation.

References and further reading

Blain, K.M. & Hill, F.J. (1998) The use of inhalation sedation and local anaesthesia as an alternative to general anaesthesia for extractions in children. *British Dental Journal*, **184**(12), 608–11.

Clark, M. & Brunick, A. (2007) *Handbook of Nitrous Oxide and Oxygen Sedation.* St Louis, Mosby.

Donaldson, D. & Meechan, J.G. (1995) The hazards of chronic exposure to nitrous oxide: an update. *British Dental Journal,* **178**(3), 95–100.

Gilchrist, F., Whitters, C.J., Cairns, A.M., Simpson, M. & Hosey, M.T. (1997) Exposure to nitrous oxide in a paediatric dental unit. *International Journal of Paediatric Dentistry,* **17**(2), 116–122.

Girdler, N.M. & Sterling, P.A. (1998) Investigation of nitrous oxide pollution arising from inhalational sedation for extraction of teeth in child patients. *International Journal of Paediatric Dentistry,* **8**(2), 93–102.

Health and Safety Commission (1995) *Anaesthetic Agents: Controlling Exposure under COSHH.* London, HMSO.

Lockwood, A.J. & Yang, Y.F. (2008) Nitrous oxide inhalation anaesthesia in the presence of intraocular gas can cause irreversible blindness. *British Dental Journal,* **204**(5), 247–248.

7 Principles and practice of intravenous sedation

INTRODUCTION

Intravenous sedation is the technique of choice for most adult dental patients requiring conscious sedation. The administration of sedation agents via the intravenous (IV) route normally produces a predictable and reliable pharmacological effect. Intravenous sedation is more potent and quicker-acting than inhalation or oral sedation and is particularly effective for very anxious or phobic dental patients and for difficult surgical procedures. It produces true pharmacological sedation rather than the psycho-pharmacological sedation that is achieved with inhalation techniques.

The practice of IV sedation is technique-sensitive; it requires the ability to perform IV cannulation which, even for the experienced dental sedationist, can be a difficult technique to master. The dental clinician also has to be able to determine an appropriate end point for sedation and drug administration. The level of sedation needs to be sufficient to enable the patient to accept operative dentistry, but not so great as to present the risk of over-sedation.

The aim of this chapter is to provide the theoretical basis from which sound clinical principles and skilled practical techniques can be developed, to ensure the safe practice of IV midazolam sedation. The material can only provide a didactic background to good practice. It is essential that supervised hands-on training and competency is achieved before applying these clinical techniques to patients.

INTRAVENOUS SEDATION AGENTS

Indications and contraindications for intravenous sedation

Indications

- Suitable for most adult dental patients
- Counteracts moderate to severe dental anxiety
- Traumatic surgical procedures
- Gag reflex and swallow reflex are present
- Mild medical conditions which may be aggravated by the stress of dental treatment, e.g. mild hypertension or asthma
- Mild intellectual or physical disability, e.g. mild learning disability, cerebral palsy.

Intravenous sedation has an important role in the management of patients with severe systemic disease or moderate to severe disability, especially if it avoids the need for general anaesthesia. However, these patients do present a significant risk and IV sedation should only be undertaken in a specialist hospital environment.

Contraindications

- History of allergy to benzodiazepines
- Impaired renal or hepatic systems
- Pregnancy and breast feeding
- Severe psychiatric disease
- Drug dependency.

Other considerations

For people with severe needle phobia who are unable to accept any type of injection, inhalation or oral sedation may be an acceptable alternative. For these patients it is sometimes necessary to combine two techniques. Inhalation sedation (or even hypnosis) may be employed initially to relax the patient enough to allow venous cannulation; once the cannula has been inserted, the IV sedative can be administered and the inhalation element of the sedation switched off.

The use of IV techniques is also, to some extent, limited in patients with poor veins. This includes patients with excessive sub-cutaneous fat, whose veins are not visible, and the elderly who frequently have friable veins which are prone to damage during cannulation.

The use of IV sedation in children (under 16 years of age) should be approached with caution. Not only do children dislike needles but IV sedation agents can have an unpredictable effect. Children can lose their controlling inhibitions and become uncooperative so that, in the event of a complication, their condition can deteriorate very rapidly. Even slight over-sedation can result in significant respiratory depression and airway obstruction. Intravenous sedation in those under the age of 16 years should be undertaken only in very special circumstances and only by those appropriately trained and experienced in paediatric sedation.

Drug choice for intravenous sedation

Intravenous sedation agents should not only have the ability to depress the central nervous system to produce a state of conscious sedation, but they should also have a margin of safety wide enough to render the unintended loss of consciousness unlikely.

Modern IV sedation techniques depend almost exclusively on the benzodiazepines. Both midazolam and diazepam are suitable IV sedatives, although the pharmacokinetics of midazolam make this the preferred choice for dental sedation and the recommended drug of choice in the UK. Midazolam is presented in two concentrations: 2mg/ml in a 5ml ampoule and 5mg/ml in a 2ml ampoule. Although both presentations contain the same amount of midazolam, the 2mg/ml (5ml vials) formulation is less concentrated and easier to titrate because of the smaller volume required for the equivalent dose.

New IV agents are currently undergoing clinical trials to evaluate their application to dental sedation. The most promising new agent is propofol, a short-acting anaesthetic drug administered via a continuous infusion or using patient-controlled sedation techniques. It has an extremely rapid recovery period which is advantageous for ambulatory patients. It is not yet licensed for use in dental sedation in the UK, but it has been the subject of some extensive trials and its properties do offer several potential benefits, particularly with rcfcrcncc to patient-controlled sedation.

Clinical effects of sedation with intravenous midazolam

- Conscious sedation with acute detachment (lack of awareness of one's surroundings) for a period of 20–30 minutes after administration, followed by a period of relaxation which may last for a further hour or more
- Anterograde amnesia, i.e. loss of memory following administration of the drug

- Muscle relaxation (useful for those with cerebral palsy)
- Anticonvulsant action
- Slight cardiovascular and respiratory depression.

Advantages and disadvantages

Advantages

- Reasonably wide margin of safety between the end point of sedation and loss of consciousness or anaesthesia (although it is easy to induce sleep with moderate over-dosage)
- A satisfactory level of sedation is attained pharmacologically rather than psychologically
- Recovery occurs within a reasonable period and the patient can usually be discharged home less than two hours following completion of treatment.

Disadvantages

- May alter a patient's perception and response to pain but it does not produce any clinically useful analgesia
- For a short period after injection the laryngeal reflexes may be obtunded. Over-dosage may result in profound respiratory depression, particularly in patients with impaired respiratory function or in those who have taken other depressants, such as alcohol
- Excessively rapid IV injection can also cause significant respiratory depression and even apnoea
- May occasionally produce disinhibition, so instead of becoming more relaxed, the patient becomes more anxious and difficult to manage.

Planning for intravenous sedation

Careful planning is essential before undertaking IV sedation in dental practice. Chapter 3 has already dealt with the selection and assessment of patients for sedation. The following section will specify the personnel and equipment required to practice IV sedation both safely and effectively.

1. Personnel
Dental clinicians should not undertake sedation unless they have been appropriately trained. In the UK, this means that dentists should have received relevant postgraduate training. This involves completing a recognised course which provides both didactic and clinical training in recognised conscious sedation techniques. It is acceptable for an appropriately trained dental clinician to sedate the patient and provide dental treatment simultaneously. The dental clinician must

be assisted by a dental nurse or other person who is appropriately trained in the field of conscious sedation. They must have knowledge of the sedation drugs and specialised equipment being used, be capable of monitoring the clinical condition of the patient and understand the relevance of blood pressure and oxygen saturation readings. It is also essential that all staff are trained to assist in the event of an emergency. The assisting dental nurse must be specifically trained in sedation and resuscitation techniques, as this is not part of the core training for dental nurses. The gold standard for training is the Certificate in Dental Sedation Nursing.

2. Equipment

Dental surgery: The suitability of the dental surgery where sedation is provided needs to be assessed. Easy access and space for patients, staff and for the management of emergencies is required. There should be the facility to store sedation agents and other drugs in a locked drugs cupboard. The dental chair must have a fast-recline mechanism so that in an emergency the patient can be quickly laid supine. There should be a high-volume aspirator available (with emergency back-up) which can be used to clear the oropharynx.

Monitoring equipment: It is essential to monitor the patient's clinical condition during sedation. The following equipment is required:

- Pulse oximeter: it is mandatory to continuously measure oxygen saturation and heart rate throughout the sedation procedure
- Manual or automatic sphygmomanometer to monitor baseline blood pressure before sedation, during sedation and prior to the patient being discharged.

Emergency equipment and drugs: Appropriate emergency equipment and drugs must also be available (detailed in Chapter 8). It is particularly important to have the facility to provide supplemental oxygen via a nasal cannula or a face-mask and an additional device with which to give positive pressure ventilation. The emergency equipment required for sedation is identical to that which should be stocked in any dental practice; the only additional item required for undertaking benzodiazepine sedation is the reversal agent, flumazenil (trade name Anexate®). This is presented as a clear liquid in 500mcg ampoules.

Recovery facility: Ideally there should be a separate recovery area where the patient can sit quietly and privately following sedation. A pulse oximeter and blood pressure monitor must be available as well as oxygen and suction apparatus. An alternative is to allow the patient to recover in the dental chair but this utilises the chair for several hours and may not be possible in a busy dental practice.

Specific sedation equipment: To administer IV sedation, the following equipment is required (Figure 7.1):
- 2 × disposable 5ml graduated syringes
- 2 × 21 gauge hypodermic needles (preferably blunt)
- Tourniquet
- Surgical wipes
- Adhesive tape (or proprietary dressings)
- Indwelling teflonated 22-gauge cannula.

Figure 7.1
Equipment required for the administration of intravenous sedation agents.

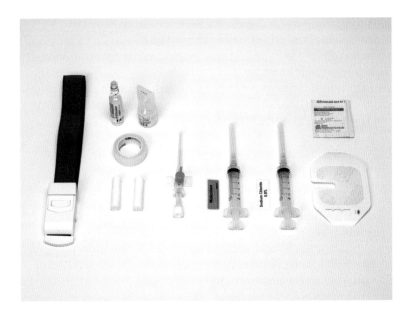

A teflonated cannula provides more secure access and is unlikely to become dislodged or blocked during limb movement. A 22-gauge cannula is the ideal size for administering IV sedatives. It readily allows the administration of modest volumes of drugs but is small enough not to cause too much discomfort on insertion.

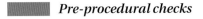 **Technique of intravenous sedation**

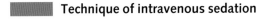 *Pre-procedural checks*

The patient scheduled for IV sedation should have undergone thorough pre-operative assessment as described in Chapter 3.

The availability of appropriate personnel and equipment should be checked before the start of each sedation session. It is helpful to use a pre-procedural checklist, such as that illustrated in Figure 7.2, to ensure that all the necessary criteria required to practise sedation safely are confirmed before the start of the session.

Each item on the list should be checked and the appropriate box ticked. Equipment should not only be available but also in good working order. Gas cylinders, and particularly oxygen supplies, must be checked to ensure that they contain a sufficient volume of gas and are not low or empty. The expiry date on all drugs should be checked to ensure that they are still valid. All the equipment required for the session should be prepared and placed discreetly out of the patient's line of vision.

Before the patient is brought into the surgery, the following information should be confirmed:

- Presence of suitable escort
- Appropriate transport home (car/taxi)
- Written consent obtained
- Medical history updated
- Routine medication taken
- Time of last meal and drink (minimum fasting time 2 hours)
- If alcohol been taken (if consumed within the previous 24 hours then treatment should be postponed).

The patient can then be escorted to the surgery and seated in the dental chair. It is important to keep waiting time to a minimum, as delays only increase the fear of an already anxious patient. The procedure for sedation and the dental treatment to be performed on that visit should be briefly re-explained to the patient. Before any sedation procedure is commenced the blood pressure should be taken and a pulse oximeter probe attached to the patient's finger or ear lobe. Once seated comfortably the chair can be reclined in preparation for venepuncture.

Venepuncture and intravenous cannulation

Establishing secure IV access is essential to the success of IV sedation. An indwelling cannula, which is present throughout the period of sedation and recovery, is mandatory for safe sedation practice. It is not acceptable to simply inject an IV sedation agent using a syringe and needle, which is then removed once the drug has been administered. Venous access is required not only for the administration of the sedation agent but also, in the event of an emergency, for the administration of a reversal agent or other emergency drug. Untoward occurrences can occur at any time during the treatment

INTRAVENOUS SEDATION TREATMENT RECORD

Affix patient identification label in box below or complete details

Surname	Patient ID No.
Forename	D.O.B. D D M M Y Y Y Y
Address	NHS No.
	Sex. Male / Female
Postcode	

Date	
Clinician - Sedationist	
- Operator	
1st Assistant	
2nd Assistant	

PRE-SEDATION CHECKLIST

1. Staff Check:

Experienced qualified assistant present?	
Another clinician/nurse within easy call?	
Clinician/assistant know emergency procedure?	

2. Emergency and Monitoring Equipment Check:

Site of Emergency Equipment known	
Oxygen - emergency/routine	
Suction - fixed/mobile - back up	
Positive pressure ventilating bag	
Sphygmomanometer - manual/automatic	
Pulse oximeter	
ECG/defibrillator	
Emergency drugs - flumazenil	

3. Sedation Equipment Check:

Midazolam, sodium chloride (drug, concn, exp date)	
22g cannulae, 5ml syringes, green needles, labels (x2)	
Tourniquet, alcohol wipe, micropore tape, stopwatch	

4. Patient Check:

Patient /parent understands what is planned	
Written consent obtained	
Medical history check	
Normal medication taken	
Last meal/drink/alcohol (Fasting - give-glucose) (Alcohol - postpone)	
Escort and transport	

Figure 7.2 Pre-operative checklist for intravenous sedation including information about the emergency equipment, intravenous sedation equipment and patient details.

appointment, so it is essential that once venous access has been established the cannula should remain *in situ* until the patient is discharged.

Teflon® is minimally irritant to veins and, due to its low adhesive surface, the cannula rarely blocks during short procedures. In addition it can bend during limb movement and once in place it will rarely become dislodged.

There are two main sites of venous access for the purposes of dental sedation, the dorsum of the hand and the antecubital fossa.

***Dorsum of the hand*:** The dorsum of the hand has a variable network of veins which drain into the cephalic and basilic veins of the forearm (Figure 7.3 and Chapter 2, Figure 2.5). These veins provide the first choice for establishing venous access as they are accessible, superficial, clearly visible in most patients, stabilised by underlying bones of the hand, and are distant from vital structures.

The disadvantage of the dorsal veins of the hand, is that they are poorly tethered and tend to move during the insertion of a cannula if the skin is not held sufficiently taught. The dorsal veins of the hand are also subject to peripheral vasoconstriction in cold weather and in patients who are very anxious. Vasoconstriction can usually be reversed by warming the hand in a bowl of warm water prior to venepuncture. The back of the hand can also be somewhat painful to puncture and consideration should be given to the use of a topical local anaesthetic agent such as EMLA® or AMETOP®, particularly in patients who are anxious about the cannulation procedure.

***Antecubital fossa*:** The second choice for venous access is in the larger veins of the antecubital fossa. (Chapter 2, Figure 2.6)

The two main veins of the forearm, the cephalic and basilic veins, pass the lateral and medial aspects of the antecubital fossa respectively. A further vein (the median vein) originates in the deep tissue of the forearm and divides to join the cephalic

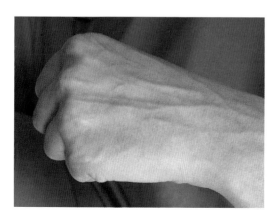

Figure 7.3
Dorsum of the hand, showing the network of superficial veins.

and basilic veins at the antecubital fossa. Any of these veins can be used for establishing venous access. However, it is important to note that the brachial artery and the median nerve also pass through the antecubital fossa on its inner aspect, medial to the biceps tendon (aponeurosis). Venepuncture and cannulation ideally should be restricted to the lateral aspect of the antecubital fossa, using the cephalic or median cephalic veins, to avoid accidental damage to vital structures.

The antecubital has the advantage of having veins which are usually large and well tethered. If not readily visible they can usually be palpated. The main disadvantage of the antecubital fossa is the proximity of important structures and the movement of the elbow joint. The use of an arm board to stabilise an extended arm can be useful.

If veins are not suitable on either the dorsum of the hand or the antecubital fossa, then the patient should be referred to a more experienced practitioner. It is possible to use the large vein lateral to the radial artery as it runs from the wrist over the radius or the great saphenous vein of the foot as it passes over the medial malleolus. However, these veins are not suitable for the inexperienced practitioner.

The key to successful venepuncture and cannulation is careful preparation of the site and a well-practised technique. Many dental clinicians see venepuncture as the most difficult part of the sedation technique to master. It is recommended that practitioners gain practical experience on mannequin arms or on willing colleagues, before attempting to cannulate anxious patients who are unlikely to tolerate multiple unsuccessful attempts at venepuncture.

Cannulation process

1. The patient should, where possible, be laid supine to minimise the chance of a vasovagal attack during venepuncture and to maximise the venous return from the extremities.
2. A suitable vein should be selected and a tourniquet placed about 10cm above that site. The dental clinician should then wait until the vein starts to become tense and filled with blood, which may take one or two minutes. The process can be accelerated by repeated clenching of the fist, thereby pumping blood into the obtunded vein. Gentle tapping of the skin over the vein often helps to make it more prominent, a process sometimes referred to as 'superficialisation'. Lowering the limb below the level of the heart will also increase venous filling.

   With difficult veins, it may be possible to get better filling by using a sphygmomanometer cuff inflated to midway between diastolic and systolic pressure. Hot towels can also be applied to the skin to encourage vasodilatation. Adequate preparation of the vein is the key to successful venepuncture and only when the vein is sufficiently full should penetration be attempted.

3. The skin should be cleaned with water or a suitable antiseptic, such as isopropyl alcohol. The latter tends to cause pain on injection unless it has completely evaporated and there is no scientific evidence that the use of alcohol is of any real benefit.

4. The skin is then tensed and the cannula inserted at an angle of around 10–15° (Figure 7.4).

It is passed through the skin and into the underlying vein for a distance of around 1cm. Skillful phlebotomists view venepuncture as a two-stage process, initially penetrating the skin and subsequently the vein. A small flashback of blood indicates correct localisation of the cannula in the lumen of the vein (Figure 7.5).

If no flashback is seen, then the cannula is still in the subcutaneous tissues and needs to be carefully advanced

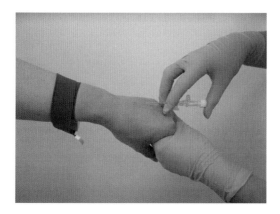

Figure 7.4
Insertion of the cannula. The skin is held taught and the cannula angled at 10–15 degrees to enter the vein.

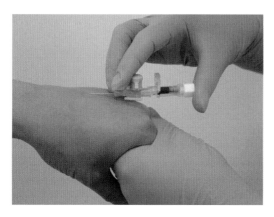

Figure 7.5
A small flashback of blood confirms that the cannula is in the lumen of the vein.

forward or laterally through the vein wall. Once a flashback of blood is visible, the teflon part of the cannula is advanced up to its hub, leaving the insertion needle static. It is better to move the teflonated section forward rather than the needle backwards as this runs a greater risk of the cannula becoming extra-venous (Figure 7.6).

5. The needle is removed completely and a cap is removed from it so that it can be placed on the aperture of the cannula. To avoid blood spilling onto the patient, pressure should then be applied just proximal to the vein where the cannula is situated.

6. Finally, the extra-venous section of the cannula is fixed securely in place, using non-allergenic surgical tape or proprietary dressing (Figure 7.7).

7. The correct positioning and patency of the cannula may be tested by administering 2–3ml of 0.9% saline intravenously (Figure 7.8).

If the cannula is sited in the lumen of the vein, the saline will pass easily into the general circulation. In contrast, if the

Figure 7.6
As the needle is withdrawn a further flashback of blood is seen within the cannula tube.

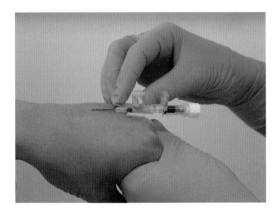

Figure 7.7
The cannula is fixed in place. Special fixing plasters or micropore tape may be used.

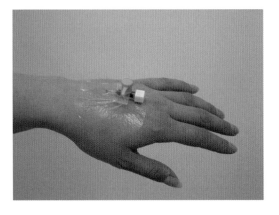

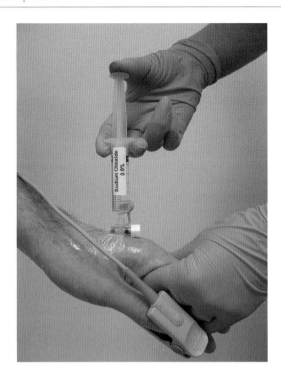

Figure 7.8
The position of the cannula is checked by injecting 2ml of 0.9% saline.

cannula has come out of the vein and is in the sub-cutaneous tissues, the saline will pool and a small lump will appear under the skin (tissuing). If this happens the cannula should be removed and reinserted at another site. The patient may feel a cold sensation moving up the arm when saline is administered into a correctly positioned cannula. If, however, there is a complaint of pain radiating down the arm, the injection must be stopped as this indicates accidental arterial cannulation.

Titration of sedation agent

The syringe containing the prepared drug (midazolam 10mg in 5ml) is attached to the delivery port of the cannula (Figure 7.9).

The patient is warned that they will begin to feel relaxed and sleepy over the next 10 minutes. The first increment of 1mg (0.5ml) midazolam is injected slowly over 15 seconds, followed by a pause for 1 minute. Further doses of 1mg are delivered, with an interval of 1 minute between increments, until the level of sedation is judged to be adequate. The aim of IV sedation, is to titrate incremental doses of drug according to the patient's response. The dental clinician should keep talking to the patient whilst carefully watching for the effects of sedation as well as any adverse reactions, especially respiratory depression. The sedation end point is reached when several specific signs of sedation are apparent. These signs include:

Figure 7.9
Titration of the sedation agent, midazolam at a rate of 1mg/min.

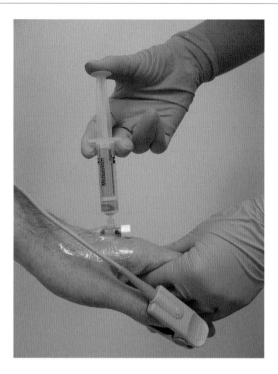

1. Slurring and slowing of speech
2. Relaxed demeanour
3. Delayed response to commands
4. Willingness to undergo treatment
5. Positive Eve's sign
6. Verill's sign.

Eve's sign is a test of motor co-ordination. The patient is requested to touch the tip of their nose with their finger. A sedated patient will be unable to accurately perform this simple task and usually touches the top lip (Figure 7.10).

Verill's sign occurs when there is ptosis or drooping of the upper eyelid, to an extent that it lies approximately half way across the pupil. These signs of sedation are not exclusive and often only two or three are present in an individual. They do, however, give some objective indication of an adequate level of sedation.

The essential criterion for conscious sedation is that communication is maintained with the patient and there are responses to the clinician's commands. Determining an appropriate end point for sedation is often difficult but depends on the ability of the dental clinician to recognise specific signs and to maintain a rapport with the patient. There is considerable variation in the dose required to produce adequate sedation between individual patients, and even

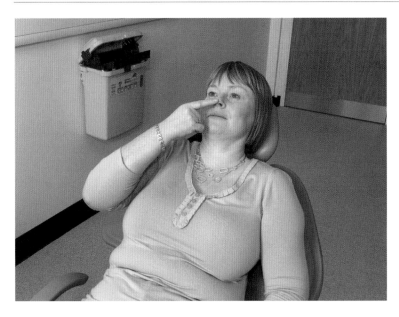

Figure 7.10
Inability to touch the tip of the nose with the forefinger indicates loss of motor co-ordination and is known as Eve's sign.

between different sessions for the same patient. Factors such as the extent of dental fear, concurrent drug therapy, the amount of sleep the previous night and the level of stress at home, are so variable that it is impossible to predict how much drug will be required for a specific patient on a certain day. This is why careful titration of the dose of sedation agent, in response to specific signs, is so important for the practice of safe sedation. If drug dose was to be based on weight only, then numerous patients would become either over- or under-sedated. When the patient is judged to be appropriately sedated, the syringe containing the sedation drug is removed and the cannula flushed through with 2–3ml of 0.9% saline. No further increments of drug are given when a standardised technique is adopted.

Clinical and electromechanical monitoring

The clinical condition of the patient must be continuously monitored throughout the sedation session. This involves the use of both clinical and electromechanical techniques.

Clinical monitoring

- Patency of the patient's airway
- Pattern of respiration
- Pulse
- Skin colour
- Level of consciousness.

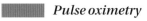 *Electromechanical monitoring*

- Pulse oximetry
- Blood pressure.

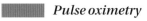 *Pulse oximetry*

Pulse oximetry is a technique which measures the patient's arterial oxygen saturation and pulse rate from a probe attached to the finger or ear lobe (Figure 7.11). This should be recorded prior to commencing drug titration and throughout treatment and recovery.

Figure 7.11
The pulse oximeter measures the patient's arterial oxygen saturation and heart rate using a finger or ear lobe probe.

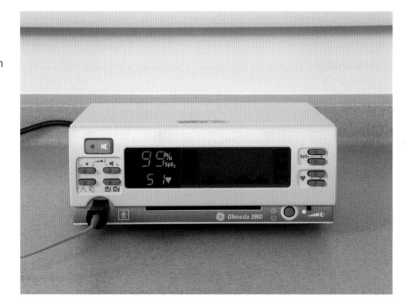

The oximeter works by measuring and comparing the absorption of two different wavelengths of red and infrared light by the arterial blood. The colour of the blood changes according to the degree of oxygen saturation and this in turn affects the absorption spectrum. By calculating the relative absorption of the two wavelengths the oximeter can precisely calculate oxygen saturation.

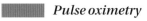 **Management of oxygen desaturation**

Oxygen saturation is an excellent monitor of both respiratory and cardiovascular function. Patients undergoing sedation should always have an oxygen saturation well above 90%. If the saturation drops below this level it is an indication of inhibited

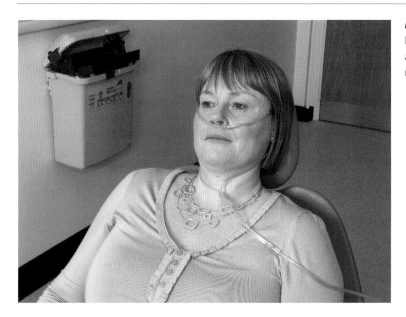

Figure 7.12
Nasal oxygen is administered via a nasal cannula.

respiratory or cardiovascular activity. The cause should be promptly investigated and corrected. The most common causes of oxygen desaturation during sedation are slight respiratory depression, breath holding or over-sedation. The problem is usually rectified by asking the patient to take a few deep breaths. If the saturation remains below 90%, supplemental oxygen should be administered via a nasal cannula at a rate of 2–4 litres/minute (Figure 7.12).

If the patient's saturation still does not rise, then the most likely cause is over-sedation. In such cases the sedation should be reversed with flumazenil.

The pulse oximeter is essentially an early warning device. It will indicate an initial problem which, with swift intervention, can be corrected before the situation becomes more serious. It should be remembered that the pulse oximeter is not infallible. Correct functioning of the equipment can be affected by excessive movement, pigmented skin, nail varnish and fluorescent or bright lights. Aberrant values should always be confirmed by clinical observation of the patient.

Pulse oximeter alarm

Pulse oximeters have an audible alarm which is activated when the saturation or pulse rate drops below a specific threshold. For routine IV sedation, the alarm should be set to sound if the saturation drops below 90% or the pulse goes below 50 or above 120. Bradycardia may indicate a vasovagal attack, vagal stimulation or hypoxia. Tachycardia usually results from inadequate analgesia and pain control. Any values outside the accepted range, should result in immediate cessation of dental treatment followed by investigation and prompt rectification of the cause.

Blood pressure monitoring

Blood pressure monitoring throughout sedation is recommended. The blood pressure should be taken immediately before IV sedation is administered, to provide a baseline value, at regular intervals during sedation and before the patient is discharged. Most hypertensive patients will have been picked up at the assessment appointment and referred for medical opinion. Some elevation of blood pressure is to be expected in anxious dental patients but if values are excessive (higher than 160/95) then sedation should be postponed until a later date. Blood pressure measuring need only be repeated during treatment if there is a concern over the clinical condition of the patient or in the event of an emergency. Blood pressure can be taken using either a manual sphygmomanometer or an automatic blood pressure machine (Figure 7.13).

It should be remembered that simple observation of the patient's clinical status is the most important type of monitoring. Although pulse oximetry is mandatory, it should not detract the dental surgeon and the dental nurse from continuously assessing the patient's clinical condition.

Figure 7.13
The patient's blood pressure is most easily monitored before, during and after treatment using an electromechanical blood pressure machine.

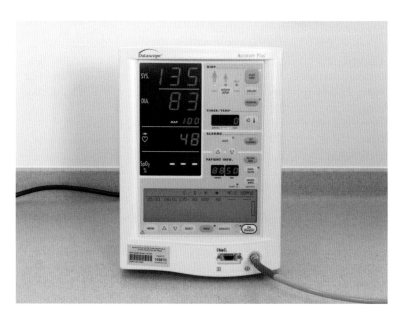

Dental treatment

The administration of local analgesia and start of operative dentistry can begin as soon as the patient has reached the appropriate level of sedation. A simple way to assess the end point of sedation is to ask the patient if he/she is comfortable for treatment to begin. Approximately 30–40 minutes of operating time is usually available following a single administration, and treatment should be planned so that it can be readily completed in this time. It is good practice to undertake traumatic procedures, such as bone removal and cavity preparation, at the beginning of the session whilst the patient is in a state of acute detachment. After 30–40 minutes the effect of sedation starts to wear off and co-operation may be reduced. This is the time to concentrate on simple procedures such as suturing or carving restorations.

Intravenous sedation using a single benzodiazepine produces no analgesia, so it is essential to provide effective pain control during dental procedures. This should include the use of both topical analgesia and sufficient quantities of local anaesthetic. Sedated patients will still respond to pain, although their response will be reduced. The muscle relaxant effect of sedation makes it difficult for patients to keep their mouths open during treatment. A mouth prop can improve access for the dental surgeon and make treatment more comfortable for the patient. It must never be an excuse, however, for failing to maintain conversation with patients and checking that their responses to instructions remain intact.

During sedation, the gag reflex is significantly diminished, and immediately following drug administration the laryngeal reflexes may also be reduced. The airway must be protected from any obstruction and this is best achieved by high volume aspiration. When small instruments are used, a rubber dam or a butterfly sponge must be inserted to protect against foreign bodies accidentally falling into the airway. Great care should be exercised when extracting teeth in the sedated patient. Use good suction to prevent segments of crowns, roots or amalgam entering the pharynx.

Recovery

At the end of the dental procedure the patient is slowly returned to the upright position over a period of several minutes. They are then transferred to the recovery area and placed in a comfortable chair or trolley. Patients should not be moved from the dental chair until they can walk with minimal assistance. Whilst in the recovery area the patient should be

Figure 7.14
Following treatment the
patient is escorted to the
recovery area where
monitoring continues
until discharge.

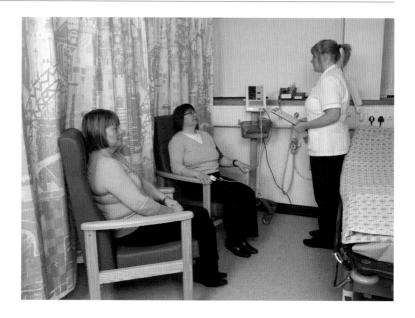

Figure 7.14
Following treatment the patient is escorted to the recovery area where monitoring continues until discharge.

under the direct supervision of the dental team or their escort (Figure 7.14).

At least one hour should have elapsed since the last increment of drug was administered before patients can be assessed for discharge. Discharge criteria include:
- Ability to walk in a straight line unassisted
- Speech no longer slurred
- Oxygen saturation back to baseline
- Blood pressure restored to near baseline
- Presence of suitable escort.

When the dental clinician determines that patients are ready to leave they should be discharged into the care of their escort who must be given full spoken and written instructions about their post-operative care (Figure 7.15).

The following advice should be provided:
- Rest quietly at home for the rest of the day
- For the next 24 hours, they should refrain from
  - Driving
  - Drinking alcohol
  - Operating machinery or domestic appliances
  - Signing legal documents
  - Making Internet transactions.

The venous cannula should remain *in situ* until just before the patient is discharged. It should be taken out by carefully removing the surgical tape or dressing and withdrawing the cannula (Figure 7.16). Firm pressure is then maintained with a

DEPARTMENT OF SEDATION

INSTRUCTIONS FOR PATIENTS AND THEIR
ESCORTS FOLLOWING TREATMENT UNDER SEDATION

This instruction sheet should be followed by the patient under the supervision of the person who has assumed responsibility for the patient's care.

Following your treatment under sedation you will be discharged home under the care of your escort. You should rest at home and reduce your activity for the next 24 hours. You are likely to feel drowsy, disorientated and forgetful for the rest of the day as the effect of the sedation takes time to wear off. You may also experience some bruising of your arm where the sedative agent was given.

It is very important that you observe the following instructions:

1. Your escort must take you home preferably by private car rather than by public transport and arrange for you to be looked after by a responsible adult for the next 24 hours.

2. You MUST NOT drive any vehicle, operate any machinery or use any domestic appliance for 24 hours following sedation.

3. You MUST NOT drink any alcohol, return to work, make any important decisions or sign any legal documents for 24 hours after sedation.

4. You should take any medicines you have been prescribed at the usual times unless instructed to the contrary.

5. If you are worried or have any problems following your treatment please telephone the Sedation Unit from 8.30am to 5.00pm, or at all other times, contact NHS Direct for advice.

If you follow these instructions you should have a pleasant and uneventful recovery from your treatment under sedation.

Figure 7.15 Written post-operative instructions are given to the patient and their escort prior to discharge.

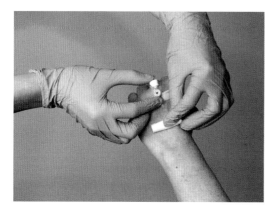

Figure 7.16 The cannula is removed just before the patient is discharged.

cotton wool roll on the venepuncture site for several minutes to prevent haematoma formation. If significant bleeding occurs when the cannula is removed it can also be helpful to elevate the arm for a period of two to three minutes. The patient should always be advised that there may be bruising at the cannulation site for several days after treatment.

Sedation records

Every sedation episode should be carefully documented in the patient notes. It can be helpful to use a printed sheet to record details of the sedation provided (Figure 7.17).

The following should be recorded prior to drug administration:

- Operating dentist and assisting dental nurse(s)
- Intravenous drug used
- Drug expiry date and batch number
- Time of first and final increment
- Total dose administered
- Size of the venous cannula
- Site of cannulation.

Although the patient is continuously monitored during sedation it is good practice to record the monitoring data at 5 minute intervals:

- Oxygen saturation
- Blood pressure
- Heart rate
- Respiration rate.

The more advanced pulse oximeters will do this automatically and provide a printout of the results. The dental treatment provided should also be documented in the normal way.

At the end of the session a note should be made about the level of sedation, operating conditions and any difficulties encountered. This information will be useful when the patient re-attends for the next sedation appointment.

Finally, information about the recovery and discharge of the patient should be recorded including:

- Oxygen saturation
- Blood pressure
- Ability to walk unassisted
- Availability of escort
- Removal of cannula
- Post-operative instructions issued to patient and escort.

The record sheet should be attached to the patient notes, along with the consent form, so that there is a complete record of the

PROCEDURAL RECORD

Intravenous Drug	Expiry Date	Batch Number	Time of Increments Initial Final	Total Dose Adminstered

Venous Access	Site			
	Canula			

Monitoring Record

Time	Oxygen Saturation	Pulse	Respiration Rate	Blood Pressure	Induction/Treatment Recovery
Continue on additional sheet					
Continue on additional sheet					

Recovery and Discharge	
Recovery with escort/nurse	
Assessment of fitness for discharge	
Written post-sedation instructions to escort & patient	
Cannula removed	
Clinician's approval to discharge	
Names of discharging - clinician - nurse	
Time of discharge	

Signature of clinician	

Figure 7.17 The patient should be monitored throughout their treatment and all information entered on the sedation treatment form.

treatment appointment. The sheet should be signed by the dental clinician and assisting dental nurse.

Complications of intravenous sedation

The complications of sedation are discussed fully in Chapter 8 and are better avoided than confronted. Good preparation is the key to reducing the incidence of complications.

Intravenous sedation is very safe, provided that it is practised on carefully selected patients, in proper facilities, by appropriately trained dental clinicians. The incidence of mortality associated with IV sedation in dentistry in the UK is extremely small. Potentially serious complications such as drug interactions, over-sedation, unconsciousness and respiratory depression are largely avoidable by careful patient selection and the use of a sound and appropriate sedation technique.

Nevertheless, IV sedation does give rise to significant minor morbidity such as haematoma at the cannulation site, and post-operative dizziness, nausea and headache.

These minor sequelae are difficult to avoid completely and are, for the most part, accepted side effects of either the sedation technique or the sedation agent. Patients should be warned of the possibility of such problems and dental surgeons should continually review their techniques to minimise the risk of any complication.

References and further reading

Dickenson, A.J. & Avery, B.S. (1995) A survey of in-dwelling intravenous cannula use in general dental practice. *British Dental Journal*, **179**(3), 89–92.

Hunter, K.M., Zacharias, M., Parkinson, R. & Luyk, N.H. (1994) Effect of flumazenil on the recovery from intravenous midazolam. *New Zealand Dental Journal*, **90**(399), 9–12.

Matsuki, Y., Ichinohe, T. & Kaneko, Y. (2007) Amnesia for electric dental pulp stimulation and picture recall test under different levels of propofol or midazolam sedation. *Acta Anaesthesiologica Scandinavica*, **51**(1), 16–21.

Oei-Lim, L.B., Vermeulen-Cranch, D.M.E. & Bouvey-Berends, E.C.M. (1991) Conscious sedation with propofol in dentistry. *British Dental Journal*, **170**(9), 340–342.

Read-Ward, G. (1990) Intravenous sedation in general dental practice: why oximetry? *British Dental Journal*, **168**(9), 368–369.

Stephens, A.J. (1993) Intravenous sedation for handicapped dental patients: a clinical trial of midazolam and propofol. *British Dental Journal*, **175**(1), 20–25.

8 Complications and emergencies

▓▓▓▓ INTRODUCTION

Sedation in dentistry has an excellent safety record. If
intravenous (IV), inhalation or oral sedation is administered
correctly to carefully selected patients, by trained dental
clinicians, with appropriate facilities and support, then the
incidence of untoward problems should be very low. However,
complications can and do occur and it is essential that all
members of the dental team practising sedation be trained
and regularly updated in the management of sedation-related
complications and medical emergencies. Where sedation is
being carried out, it is essential that the appropriate emergency
equipment and drugs are available, ready for immediate use
should the need arise.

To ensure the safe practice of conscious sedation, dental
clinicians and their assisting staff must be suitably qualified
and experienced. Postgraduate training in sedation is
mandatory. As a minimum requirement, training should cover
the theoretical and practical aspects of conscious sedation and
provide hands-on supervised clinical experience.

By definition, a true emergency is one which occurs without
warning and which could not reasonably have been foreseen.
Medical emergencies can affect anyone, at any time,
irrespective of whether they are at home, at work, walking
down the street or in a dental surgery.

Many sedation-related complications are predictable and
thus emergencies should be avoidable by good planning and
skilful technique. The need for careful and thorough pre-
sedation patient assessment cannot be over-emphasised. The
fitness of each patient to undergo treatment under sedation,
and thus the risk which sedation presents to the patient, must
be individually assessed. If any aspect of the medical history
suggests a potential problem, then expert advice should be
sought, either from the patient's medical practitioner or by
referral to a hospital specialist. Dental treatment requiring

sedation is never so urgent as to put the patient's life at risk from inadequate assessment and planning.

Adherence to the principles of good sedation practice should minimise the incidence of problems. However, despite careful preparation and technique, complications and emergencies can still arise. This chapter will discuss the emergency equipment and drugs required when practising sedation, the aetiology, clinical features and management of specific sedation-related problems and medical emergencies and the prevention and treatment of local complications.

In July 2006, the Resuscitation Council (UK) published guidelines specific to dental practice dealing with the management of medical emergencies and resuscitation. The guiding principles of this document state:

Medical emergencies can happen at any time in dental practice. If you employ, manage or lead a team, you should make sure that:
- There are arrangements for at least two people to be available to deal with medical emergencies when treatment is planned to take place.
- All members of staff, not just the registered team members, know their role if a patient collapses or there is another kind of medical emergency.
- All members of staff who might be involved in dealing with a medical emergency are trained and prepared to deal with such an emergency at any time and practise together regularly in a simulated emergency so they know exactly what to do.

This chapter will consider the management of general medical emergencies and specific sedation-related emergencies with reference to the adult patient. With regard to the management of children, readers should access the Resuscitation Council (UK) website and their own National Drug Formulary for paediatric drug doses.

EMERGENCY EQUIPMENT

It is recommended by the Resuscitation Council (UK) that the equipment used for any medical emergency or cardiopulmonary arrest should be standardised throughout general dental practices. All clinical areas should have immediate access to resuscitation drugs, equipment for airway management and an automated external defibrillator (AED). Staff must be familiar with the location of all resuscitation equipment within their working area. The necessary equipment is illustrated in Table 8.1.

Table 8.1	Emergency equipment essential for the provision of conscious sedation

- Portable oxygen cylinder (D size) with pressure-reduction valve and flow meter

- Oxygen face mask with tubing

- Basic set of oropharyngeal airways (sizes 1, 2, 3, 4)

- Pocket mask with oxygen port

- Self-inflating bag and mask apparatus with oxygen reservoir and tubing (1 litre size bag)

- Variety of well fitting adult and child face masks for attaching to self-inflating bag

- Portable suction with appropriate suction catheters and tubing, e.g. the Yankauer sucker

- Single-use sterile syringes and needles

- 'Spacer' device for inhaled bronchodilators

- Automated blood glucose measurement device

- Automated External Defibrillator

Airway management

Independent oxygen supply

The most important piece of emergency equipment (or drugs) is an independent oxygen supply. A full oxygen cylinder, size D (340 litres) or size E (680 litres), which is independent of any routine oxygen supply, should be available for an emergency. The cylinder must have a reducing valve, key, flow meter, tubing and suitable connectors. It must be readily attachable to a face mask, nasal cannula and ambu-bag or pocket-mask. It is essential that the level of oxygen in the cylinder is checked before the start of a sedation session and the cylinder should be turned on ready for immediate use if necessary. Cylinders should be stored on a portable trolley so that they can be used anywhere in the practice.

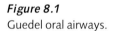 *Airway adjuncts*

A selection of Guedel oral airways must be available (Figure 8.1).
These are used to maintain a patent airway in an unconscious
patient. The commonest cause of airway obstruction in the
unconscious patient is caused by the tongue falling back onto
the anterior wall of the pharynx. This problem can usually be
relieved by placing the patient in the lateral recovery position
or by pulling the mandible forwards using the chin lift or jaw
thrust.

A simple means of assisting airway maintenance is to insert
a Guedel oral airway. This sits over the back of the tongue,
preventing it falling posteriorly into the pharynx. Air can then
pass freely in and out via the hollow airway lumen. The oral
airway requires careful insertion to ensure that the tongue
is not pushed backwards upon insertion. For this reason it is
inserted upside down as far as the back of the hard palate, then
it is turned over into the correct orientation. The Guedel airway
can only be used in an unconscious patient. It will be forcefully
ejected once the patient regains consciousness and the
pharyngeal reflexes return.

Nasopharyngeal airways are very useful in a semi-conscious
patient. They are designed to be inserted into the nasal
passageway to secure an open airway. The correct size airway
is chosen by measuring the device on the patient: the device
should reach from the patient's nostril to the earlobe or the
angle of the jaw. The outside of the tube is lubricated with a
water-based lubricant so that it enters the nose more easily.

Figure 8.1
Guedel oral airways.

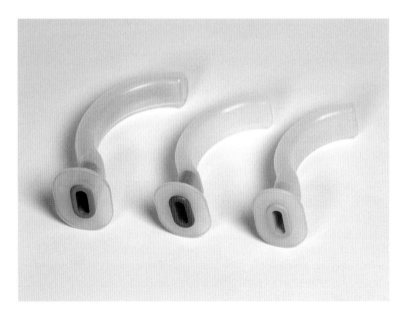

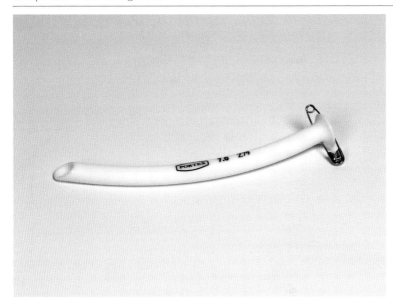

Figure 8.2
Nasal airway.

The device is inserted until the flared end rests against the nostril (Figure 8.2).

Intermittent positive pressure device

A ventilating device for administering oxygen under intermittent positive pressure is an essential piece of equipment. This is used to support ventilation in a patient who becomes significantly hypoxic, apnoeic or has a respiratory arrest. The classic example is the 'ambu-bag' which consists of a self-inflating bag, with an oxygen attachment, one-way valve and face mask (Figure 8.3).

When attached to an oxygen supply this bag will deliver approximately 40% oxygen in air. A higher percentage of oxygen, up to 80%, can be administered by attaching an oxygen reservoir bag to the main self-inflating bag. The ambu-bag requires two people to operate it efficiently, one to hold the mask on the face to maintain a good seal and to support the airway, the other to squeeze the bag and ventilate the patient. It is possible to use the ambu-bag single-handedly but it can be difficult to perform these tasks simultaneously. Another example of an intermittent positive pressure device is the simple pocket-mask with an oxygen attachment (Figure 8.4).

This is easier to use by a single person than the ambu-bag because the manual effort is aimed at holding the mask in position and maintaining the airway. Ventilation is achieved by the practitioner actually breathing into the mask. The percentage of oxygen delivered is less than that achieved with

Figure 8.3
Ambu-bag with reservoir
bag.

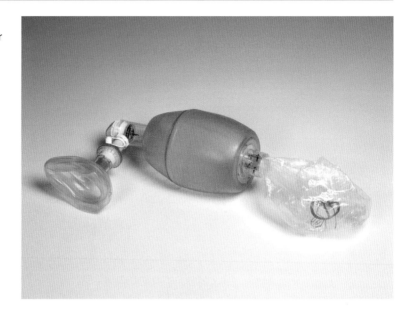

Figure 8.4
Pocket mask used for
giving rescue breaths
during cardiopulmonary
resuscitation.

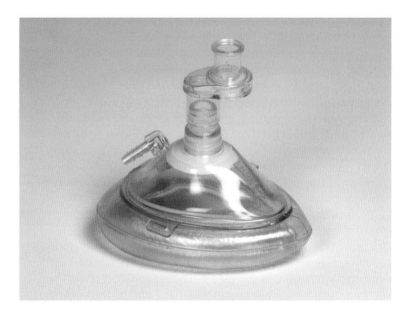

an ambu-bag, but the device is easier to operate and may be
more efficient than an improperly used ambu-bag.

Suction equipment

Portable suction equipment (preferably totally independent of
the main suction supply) should always be available. Although
the laryngeal reflexes in a sedated patient are intact they do

have a reduced gag reflex and less ability to remove vomit or foreign bodies from the mouth. The suction apparatus should be portable so that it can be used in the recovery area or any other part of the dental practice. It should also be independent of the power supply so it will still function if there is a power failure. Manual suction devices are available which do not require a power source.

DRUG ADMINISTRATION

A list of recommended emergency drugs is shown in Table 8.2. It is essential that the dental surgeon understands the indication for each drug and how it is administered. There is little point in stocking a drug if it cannot be used appropriately.

A range of disposable syringes (5ml and 2ml) and needles (23g) should be available to administer parenteral drugs, intramuscularly or intravenously, in an emergency. A selection of teflonated cannulae (20g) should also be kept in the emergency stock so that additional venous access can be gained should the original sedation cannula become blocked or dislodged (see Figure 8.5).

Table 8.2	Emergency drugs, doses and application

- Oxygen

- Epinephrine injection (1:1000, 1mg/ml)

- Hydrocortisone hemisuccinate (100mg/2ml)

- Chlorphenamine maleate (10mg/1ml)

- Oral glucose solution / tablets / gel / powder

- Glucagon injection 1mg

- Glyceryl trinitrate (GTN) spray (400micrograms / dose)

- Salbutamol aerosol inhaler (100micrograms / actuation)

- Aspirin dispersable (300mg)

- Midazolam 5mg/ml

- Flumazenil (500ug/5ml)

Figure 8.5
Example of emergency
drugs .

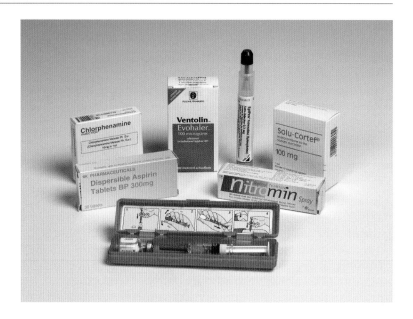

Oxygen

The most important 'drug' for any dental practice to stock is
oxygen. This is the first and, in many cases, the only substance
which is required in an emergency situation. It is of particular
importance in sedation because almost all sedation agents
produce some degree of respiratory depression. The normal
concentration of oxygen in the air is 21%. By administering
100% oxygen from a cylinder, via a nasal cannula or face
mask, the inspired percentage of oxygen can be significantly
increased. This will help to compensate for the slight
desaturation that can occur as a result of mild respiratory
depression. The administration of 100% oxygen is also an
essential first step in the management of nearly all medical
emergencies.

Epinephrine

Epinephrine at a concentration of 1mg/1ml (1 in 1000 dilution)
is required for the treatment of anaphylaxis. Epinephrine is
administered either intramuscularly or subcutaneously. It
must never be delivered via the IV route in general dental
practice.

Hydrocortisone hemisuccinate

Hydrocortisone hemisuccinate (100mg/2ml) should be stocked
for the management of an adrenal crisis and anaphylaxis.

It is presented as an anhydrous hydrocortisone powder and a separate ampoule of water. The two are mixed together immediately before administration. Hydrocortisone can be delivered intramuscularly, subcutaneously or intravenously. If administered via the IV route the 100mg hydrocortisone powder should be diluted into 10ml of water and given slowly.

Chlorphenamine maleate

Chlorphenamine maleate (10mg/1ml) is an antihistamine which should be available for the management of more minor allergic reactions. It is presented in solution and is administered intramuscularly or intravenously. Antihistamines have limited value in the management of anaphylaxis since.

Glucose or dextrose

Glucose or dextrose tablets or gel should be available for use in the early stages of a hypoglycaemic attack in a diabetic patient. A conscious patient should be given tablets to suck or the gel can be smoothed onto the oral mucosa. Alternatively a glucose-based drink can be given. However, if the patient's condition is deteriorating there should be no hesitation about giving IV glucose or 1mg of glucagon intramuscularly (see below).

Glucagon

Glucagon (1mg) is required if the hypoglycaemic patient loses consciousness. It is administered subcutaneously, intramuscularly or intravenously. Sterile glucose or dextrose (50ml of a 50% solution) which is delivered intravenously should also be available. This acts more rapidly than glucagon but its high viscosity can make it difficult to administer through the narrow bore cannulae used to administer sedation drugs. A 25% dilution is also available and is easier to administer.

Glyceryl trinitrate

Glyceryl trinitrate tablets (0.3mg) or glyceryl trinitrate spray (0.4mg/dose) are required for the management of angina. Both tablets and spray are administered sublingually to maximise the rate of absorption.

Aspirin

Soluble aspirin tablets (300mg) should be stocked for use in the event of a myocardial infarction. Aspirin reduces platelet adhesiveness and is used to reduce the morbidity of myocardial infarction. There is good evidence that early administration improves outcomes and reduces mortality after myocardial infarction.

 Salbutamol

A salbutamol inhaler (0.1mg/dose) or a salbutamol nebuliser with nebules (2.5mg) should be available for the management of an acute asthma attack.

 Midazolam

Midazolam (10mg/2ml) is recommended for the treatment of status epilepticus, however for any patient who has already received midazolam sedation, care must be taken not to over-dose the patient.

 Flumazenil

All of the above emergency drugs should be available in a dental practice, irrespective of whether sedation is being provided or not. The only additional emergency drug which must be stocked where sedation is being practised is the benzodiazepine antagonist, flumazenil (500mg/5ml). Alongside oxygen, this is probably the most useful drug for dealing with emergencies arising as a result of over-sedation. However, it does not obviate the need for instituting basic life support procedures at the first sign of any untoward problem.

 Defibrillation

It is recommended by the Resuscitation Council (UK) that all clinical areas should have access to an automated external defibrillator (AED) (Figure 8.6). An AED will reduce mortality from cardiac arrest caused by ventricular fibrillation and pulseless ventricular tachycardia. It is considered that the availability of an AED enables dental staff to attempt defibrillation safely after appropriate training. Adult AEDs can safely be used on children over 8 years old. Some machines have paediatric pads or a mode that permits them to be 'attenuated' to make them more suitable for use in children between 1 and 8 years of age.

 SEDATION-RELATED EMERGENCIES

The treatment of patients under sedation carries a number of inherent potential risks. The key to successful management of

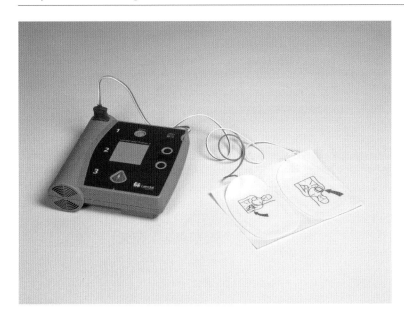

Figure 8.6
Automated external
defibrillator.

emergencies is early identification and intervention. When a
patient is being treated under sedation the dental clinician and
dental nurse should be continuously aware of the:
• Patency of the airway
• Rate and depth of breathing
• Heart rate
• Arterial oxygen saturation
• Skin colour
• Level of consciousness.

Careful clinical monitoring, supplemented with pulse
oximetry, is mandatory. At the first sign of any untoward
problem, dental treatment should immediately be terminated
and full attention must be paid to the patient's clinical status.
  Any significant alteration of clinical signs, such as a
reduction in respiration rate or pulse rate, should prompt the
dental clinician to take immediate action. For example, if a
patient becomes pale and nauseous during the induction of
sedation this may indicate an impending vasovagal attack.
Unless the patient is laid supine rapidly they will lose
consciousness. This is not the effect of the sedation drug
(although it may be compounded by it) but is a simple faint.
Careful monitoring of the patient's clinical status will alert
the dental surgeon to the early signs of an untoward problem.
Failing to observe or ignoring the signs of impending problems
and delaying management is negligent on the part of the
practitioner and may put the patient at serious risk.

The pulse oximeter can be very useful in providing an early warning of impending problems developing. For example, a drop in oxygen saturation will normally be identified by the oximeter long before any clinical signs of desaturation appear. If the dental surgeon intervenes immediately then the problem can be corrected using simple measures. Slight oxygen desaturation can be reversed by asking the patient to breath deeply or by administrating nasal oxygen. However, if the dental surgeon fails to intervene early, the problem can become difficult to manage and may even become life-threatening.

A number of complications and emergencies relate specifically to sedation. The dental clinician practising sedation must be able to distinguish between sedation-related emergencies and medical emergencies occurring in the sedated patient.

Anxiety-related problems

Exacerbation of a medical condition

Severe anxiety can also precipitate an acute exacerbation of a pre-existing medical condition, such as angina, asthma or epilepsy. Even patients with apparently well-controlled medical conditions, can deteriorate when presented with a situation which increases anxiety. Such acute medical problems may present at any stage during the sedation appointment and should be treated using the standard protocols, which are discussed later in this chapter. For most cases of pre-existing disease, appropriate precautions should have been taken to minimise the chance of precipitating an acute exacerbation.

Vasovagal attack (faint)

Patients undergoing sedation are often acutely anxious and very prone to having a vasovagal attack (faint). This usually occurs during cannulation or in the early stages of sedative drug administration. It can be largely averted by laying the patient supine before beginning the procedure. However, if a patient does become pale, clammy and nauseous then the most likely cause is vasovagal syncope. The heart rate will be rapid initially and will slow down as consciousness is lost. ***Management:*** The patient should immediately be laid flat with the legs raised and any drug administration stopped. If the patient becomes unconscious the airway should be maintained and oxygen administered via a face mask. Consciousness should be rapidly regained, although the patient may be drowsy due to the effect of any sedation agent administered prior to the faint. Severe faints, i.e. those where consciousness is lost, can also result in minor fit. This should not be confused with an epileptic attack which is progressive unlike a faint, when the shaking stops rapidly once the blood circulation to the brain has been re-established.

Respiratory depression

The most likely complication of benzodiazepine sedation is respiratory depression. This is known to occur with all benzodiazepines but it is not usually of any clinical significance and the arterial blood remains well saturated. However, excessively rapid IV administration, benzodiazepine over-dosage or adverse drug interaction can have a significant effect on the respiratory system. In addition, the very young and very old are particularly sensitive to the respiratory depressant effects of IV sedative agents. Careful patient selection, slow titration of the sedation agent and continuous clinical and electromechanical monitoring will minimise the risk.
Management: If there is any evidence of respiratory compromise this should be corrected immediately by maintaining the airway, administering oxygen and if necessary by providing assisted positive pressure ventilation. If the oxygen saturation falls and cannot be restored with simple measures, then the respiratory depressant effects of the sedation should be reversed by administering 200–500 mcg of flumazenil.

Airway obstruction – choking

Airway obstruction by aspiration of a foreign body is a potential hazard of treating patients under sedation. Sedation causes some reduction in the gag reflex and if a tooth, a piece of amalgam or a reamer is dropped to the back of the mouth the patient may find it difficult to expel the foreign body. Good airway protection using a rubber dam or a butterfly sponge and high-volume suction should avoid this problem.
Management: If a patient shows signs of mild airway obstruction they should be encouraged to cough. This will normally clear the airway and allow the patient to breath normally. Where this is not successful and more severe airway obstruction is witnessed, the rescuer should give up to five back blows between the shoulder blades with the heel of the hand. The patient should be encouraged to lean forward to assist the obstructing object to come out of the mouth. If this fails to clear the airway obstruction it will be necessary to perform up to five abdominal thrusts. Positioned behind the patient the dental clinician clasps the hands firmly around the patient's waist.

Firm pressure applied to the abdomen just below the xiphisternum will force the diaphragm up and the expired air should expel the foreign body. If the obstruction is still not cleared, continue alternating with five back blows. It should be noted that abdominal thrusts may cause internal injury or fractured ribs, it is therefore important that the patient is examined by a doctor following management of the choking episode.

Hypotension

Sedation agents will produce some level of reduction in the patient's blood pressure as a result of reduced sympathetic activity. This generally remains within safe clinical limits and requires no active intervention. However, significant hypotension may occur, where the systolic and/or diastolic pressures drop 15–20mmHg below baseline, if the patient is over-sedated or rises too quickly from the supine position.

Signs: Restlessness, disorientation, pallor, cold, clammy skin, dilated pupils.

Management: Hypotension in the sedated patient should be managed by:

1. Stopping the dental treatment and placing the patient in the supine position with the feet elevated
2. Initiating basic life support (airway, breathing, circulation)
3. Administering oxygen (3 l/min)
4. Definitive therapy:
   a. If inhalation sedation with nitrous oxide has been used, decrease the concentration
   b. If IV midazolam is being used, reverse with flumazenil
   c. Where these steps fail to manage the hypotensive episode a rapid IV infusion of 250ml solution (5% dextrose and water or 0.9% saline) will provide extra fluid volume in the cardiovascular system, leading to an increase in blood pressure
   d. Call the emergency paramedics.

Drug interactions

The use of the IV route of sedation drug administration may result in more rapid and severe drug reactions and interactions. Anaphylaxis, drug idiosyncrasy and drug interactions can all occur with IV sedation. An awareness of any previous reaction to a drug and slow incremental administration of the sedation agent and cessation of administration should any untoward problems occur, will minimise the onset and severity of drug complications. Drug interactions vary in severity and are more difficult to manage.

Management: At the first sign of any untoward reaction, the administration of the sedation agent should be stopped and the patient's clinical status should be monitored. Basic life support measures should be initiated if necessary and expert assistance summoned. A true anaphylactic reaction should be treated using the standard protocol described in the next section.

Loss of consciousness

By definition, patients undergoing conscious sedation should never lose consciousness. However, unconsciousness does sometimes occur as a direct result of sedation. It usually results from the administration of an excessive dose of sedation agent, drug idiosyncrasy or drug interaction. It may also be caused by an untoward medical emergency, totally unconnected to the sedation, such as faint cardiac arrest, diabetic coma, adrenal crisis or stroke. Sedation-related causes of unconsciousness can be avoided by obtaining a detailed drug history and by slow and careful titration of the sedation agent related to the patient's response.

Management: If the patient shows signs of over-sedation and becomes unresponsive to commands, then oxygen should be administered. If the oxygen saturation cannot be maintained at a satisfactory level the sedation should be reversed by administering flumazenil. Patients who become unconscious should be placed on their side and the airway should be maintained. Assistance must be immediately summoned and the patient monitored closely for signs of cardio-respiratory compromise. If the loss of consciousness is the result of over-sedation, the patient should regain consciousness within 2–3 minutes of receiving the reversal agent. If the patient remains unconscious then a medical cause should be suspected, identified and managed using standard protocols.

A dental clinician providing a sedation service should be competent to undertake the immediate management of sedation-related emergencies. However, there should be no hesitation to call the emergency services if there are concerns about a patient's clinical status.

MEDICAL EMERGENCIES

Medical emergencies are largely unpredictable and can occur in any patient, whether undergoing sedation or not. It requires greater vigilance to identify medical emergencies which occur during sedation and it can be difficult to distinguish them from specific sedation-related complications. Nevertheless, the clinical features and management of specific medical emergencies are the same irrespective of whether they occur in a sedated or a fully conscious patient. Every dental clinician should be able to recognise and manage a medical emergency; for the dental sedationist there is an extra duty of care.

Cardiac arrest

The most serious medical emergency is a cardiac arrest. This can occur for a variety of reasons, including as a result of hypoxia, myocardial infarction, anaphylaxis or severe hypotension. Any state which causes respiratory obstruction or apnoea will lead to respiratory arrest and ultimately, if not treated, cardiac arrest. The basic protocol for managing a cardiac arrest can be easily remembered by following the algorithm below (Figure 8.7). The recommended ratio for providing cardiac compressions and rescue breaths is at a ratio of 30:2.

There are some key factors which determine a patient's chance of recovering from a cardiac arrest, often referred to as 'the chain of survival'. The best opportunity for survival exists if each link in the chain is put into practice within minutes of the collapse occurring (Figure 8.8).

The commonest type of cardiac arrest in adults is ventricular fibrillation, therefore early defibrillation (i.e. within minutes) provides the greatest chance of survival and thus it is essential to call for an ambulance as soon as a cardiac arrest is diagnosed.

Vasovagal syncope (faint)

The most frequent cause of collapse in the dental surgery is a vasovagal attack or faint. It can be initiated by anxiety, pain, hypotension, and fatigue and occasionally fasting. Severely anxious and phobic patients undergoing sedation are especially prone to fainting. A vasovagal attack starts when a stimulus such as acute anxiety or pain produces a 'fight or flight' response. Due to vasodilatation, blood pools in the skeletal muscle and in the mesentery in the abdomen. In the absence of limb movements, venous return is reduced and the cardiac output falls. Initially this may be offset by an increase in heart rate, but if the venous return is still not restored, vagal decompensation occurs. This results in bradycardia, a reduction in cerebral blood flow and loss of consciousness.

Vasovagal syncope can largely be prevented by laying the patient supine before commencing treatment and particularly before venepuncture. If this is not possible, then the patient must be observed closely for the premonitionary signs of a

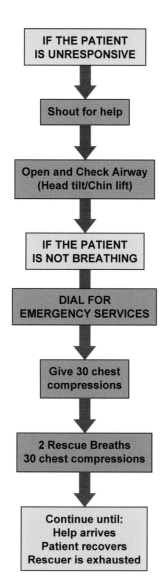

Figure 8.7
Algorithm for adult basic life support. Chest compressions and rescue breaths should be administered at a ratio of 30:2.

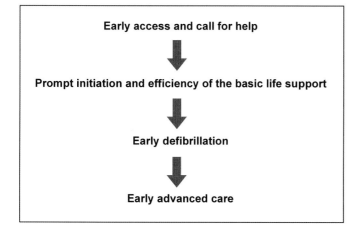

Figure 8.8
The 'chain of survival'.

vasovagal attack. If any occur, the patient must immediately be laid supine.

Signs: Pallor, nausea, perspiration on the forehead and upper lip, rapid pulse.

Management: If a patient is not immediately treated they will rapidly lose consciousness and the pulse will become slow and weak. The pulse may fall as low as 30 beats per minute. If treatment is delayed any further the patient may fit and become cyanotic. Management of a vasovagal attack includes:

- Lay the patient supine and raise the legs. Pregnant patients should be placed in the lateral position so that the weight of the foetus does not obstruct the inferior vena cava and thereby further reduce venous return
- Maintain the airway and administer oxygen via a face mask (3 l/min)
- The patient should recover rapidly
- Once consciousness has been regained reassure the patient and give a glucose drink
- If recovery is not rapid, then the diagnosis should be reconsidered, whilst the airway and oxygenation are maintained.

Sometimes it is possible to mistake vasovagal syncope for the effects of over-sedation. If a patient suddenly loses consciousness during the induction or maintenance of sedation, there should be a high index of suspicion that a vasovagal attack has occurred and appropriate treatment should be instituted.

Hypoglycaemia

Hypoglycaemia is the commonest cause of diabetic coma and can occur in patients with diabetes mellitus. It can be initiated by a missed meal, excessive anxiety or the presence of infection. All patients with diabetes mellitus undergoing dental care should be treated with caution and the dental clinician should always be alert to the possibility of hypoglycaemia.

Signs: Irritability, aggression, lack of co-operation, cold, clammy skin, drowsy and disoriented, gradual loss of consciousness despite a rapid and often full pulse.

Management:
- Whilst a patient remains conscious, they should be given glucose or dextrose drink, tablets or gel by mouth.
- If the patient becomes unconscious give 1mg glucagon intravenously, intramuscularly or subcutaneously. If the patient already has venous access give 50ml of 50% glucose or equivalent.
- Maintain airway and administer oxygen (3 l/min).

- Recovery should be rapid, whereupon consideration should be given to having the patient transferred to hospital.

Diabetic patients: If a diabetic patient undergoing IV sedation becomes unconscious, glucose should be administered immediately via the IV cannula, or intramuscular glucagon should be given, as above. If hypoglycaemia was the cause of unconsciousness, recovery will be rapid.

Anaphylaxis

The term anaphylaxis is commonly used for hypersensitivity reactions typically mediated by immunoglobulin E (IgE) in a previously sensitised individual; occasionally the recipient is unaware of his/her sensitivity. True anaphylaxis is not mediated through histamine release, although raised histamine levels are a feature of anaphylaxis. In dentistry, the most likely cause is an allergy to an antibiotic, especially penicillin or its derivatives, although milder skin-type allergies are more common. However, anaphylactic reactions can be initiated by a range of antigenic stimuli, including local anaesthetic solutions, IV drugs and latex gloves.
Signs:
- Flushing and oedema of the face and neck
- Acute breathing difficulties, with bronchospasm and wheezing
- Parasthesia around mouth and fingers
- Severe hypotension
- Rapid, weak or impalpable pulse
- Pallor and cyanosis
- Loss of consciousness.

Management: Treatment of anaphylaxis must be immediate. The patient should be laid flat with the legs raised. Epinephrine 0.5mg (1 in 1000) should be administered intramuscularly or subcutaneously. The airway should be maintained and oxygen administered. If bronchospasm persists, a further injection of 0.5mg epinephrine should be given. Expert emergency assistance should be summoned immediately and hydrocortisone sodium succinate (100mg) and chlorphenamine maleate (10–20mg) should be administered intravenously or intramuscularly.

Adrenal shock

Patients with primary or secondary adrenal disease (e.g. Addison's disease) can suffer from adrenal shock in a stressful situation. Some authorities would consider patients on long-term high-dose steroids also to be at risk. Those presenting for sedation are at particular risk because of the high level of inherent anxiety or fear. The signs of adrenal shock are pallor, a rapid weak pulse, hypotension and ultimately loss of consciousness. Treatment should commence by laying the patient flat with the head down. The airway should be maintained and oxygen delivered via a face mask. Hydrocortisone sodium succinate (100mg) should be administered intravenously or intramuscularly. If there is no improvement, further doses of hydrocortisone should be administered until 500mg has been given and the diagnosis should be reconsidered. An emergency ambulance should be summoned. A patient who is potentially at risk from adrenal shock should be given steroid cover before treatment under sedation. This will minimise the likelihood of an adrenal crisis during treatment. If the patient does become unconscious during sedation, then further hydrocortisone should be administered immediately. Patients who receive steroid therapy are at greater risk of steroid crisis and this should always be considered when a medical history is taken. The use of potent skin preparations or even steroid inhalers is frequently omitted from consideration, and the potential risk of these products needs to be highlighted.

Epilepsy

Two forms of epilepsy are generally recognised: petit mal and grand mal. The former usually results in little more than a transient loss of consciousness for a relatively short period. True epileptic fits usually occur in known epileptics who have a poorly controlled drug regimen. Fits may be precipitated by stress, anxiety and starvation and are thus more likely in patients who are undergoing sedation. The signs of an epileptic fit are loss of consciousness and rigid extended limbs, followed by jerking movements and sometimes incontinence or cyanosis. The fits are followed by a slow recovery and confusion. Treatment is aimed at protecting the patient from injury and placing them in the recovery position. The airway should be maintained and oxygen administered. If status epilepticus occurs, with persistent fitting lasting over five minutes or with signs of significant respiratory compromise, 5mg of midazolam (10mg/5ml) should be administered by slow IV injection or 5mg midazolam (10mg/2ml) by intramuscular injection, or 10mg (10mg/2ml)buccally. Theoretically, the incidence of fits occurring during benzodiazepine sedation should be low because of the anticonvulsant effect of the benzodiazepines. However, there have been a number of reports of fits arising during midazolam sedation, in epileptics. Caution should therefore be exercised when considering sedation for patients with a history of epilepsy. Fits can also occur in patients who lose consciousness for any other reason, especially those who faint and who are not immediately placed in a supine position.

Acute chest pain

Acute chest pain is usually caused by stable angina but the possibility of an acute coronary syndrome (unstable angina or myocardial infarction) should always be considered.

Stable angina results from myocardial ischaemia caused by narrowing of the coronary arteries. The demands of the heart increase during exercise, stress or hypertension and it is these situations which are most likely to precipitate an angina attack. Patients with dental anxiety undergoing sedation are more at risk. The features of an angina attack are a severe retrosternal pain radiating down the left arm and a regular pulse. Sublingual glyceryl trinitrate spray (0.4mg), should be administered, the airway should be maintained and oxygen given. If there is no relief in three minutes, the possibility of unstable angina or myocardial infarction should be considered.

Unstable angina is caused by fissuring of atheromatous plaques and subsequent platelet accumulation in a coronary artery. This results in varying degrees of occlusion of the affected artery. In myocardial infarction there is complete occlusion of a coronary artery, leading to sudden ischaemia and irreversible damage to part of the heart muscle. In myocardial infarction the patient will have severe crushing, retrosternal chest pain, which will not be relieved by use of glyceryl trinitrate. They will be pale and cyanosed, breathless and may vomit. The pulse will be weak and irregular. The patient should be allowed to find the most comfortable position to minimise the pain and this will usually be in the seated position. Patients should not be reclined unless they lose consciousness, since this increases the venous return and hence the cardiac output, thereby making more demands on the oxygen-starved myocardium. Nitrous oxide 50% with oxygen 50% (if available) should be administered to relieve pain and anxiety. Soluble aspirin (300mg) should be given orally and the emergency services should be summoned. The patient must be closely monitored for any deterioration, particularly cardiac arrest, in which case cardiopulmonary resuscitation should be initiated.

Asthma

Asthma is a very common condition which varies considerably in severity. An acute asthma attack may be precipitated by anxiety, infection, exercise or sensitivity to an allergen or irritant. The commonest signs of an asthma attack are breathlessness, with wheezing on expiration. Another presentation of asthma is of persistent coughing with progressive difficulty in breathing. In either case, the mainstay of treatment is to reassure the patient and allow them to maintain a position most comfortable for breathing. Oxygen and a salbutamol inhaler or nebuliser should be administered. If there is no improvement or if the attack turns into status asthmaticus, the emergency services should be called. Oxygenation should be maintained and hydrocortisone sodium succinate (100mg) administered intravenously or intramuscularly.

Cerebrovascular accident

A stroke is a clinical term referring to a total or partial attack of weakness on one side of the body. It may be primary (when it can be caused by cerebral haemorrhage, thrombosis or embolism) or secondary (when the primary disease is in the heart or blood vessels). The patient will often complain of a sudden headache and may have dysarthria (unclear speech) or aphasia (inability to speak). There will be some degree of hemiplegia (partial or complete paralysis of one side of the face and/or body) and there may be loss of consciousness. The airway should be maintained and oxygen administered. Respiration must be monitored and assisted ventilation commenced if breathing ceases. The emergency paramedics should be summoned.

LOCAL COMPLICATIONS

There are a number of local complications which can occur with IV sedation.

*1. Extravenous injection***:** This happens when the cannula either fails to penetrate the lumen of the vein or completely transects the vein. In both cases the cannula will become located in the subcutaneous tissues. Flushing with 0.9% saline will clearly indicate if the cannula is not in the lumen of the vein. Saline will pool subcutaneously and a lump will be visible. If this occurs the cannula should be removed and re-sited elsewhere. If there is no sign of extravasation the sedation agent can be administered. Should any sedation agent be accidentally deposited in the subcutaneous tissues, the injection should be stopped and the area massaged to disperse the drug. Small quantities of extravenous midazolam usually disperse freely and cause no residual problems. An acute inflammatory reaction may occur with extravenous injection of diazepam but it is not usually necessary to administer vasodilators. Rarely, if an excessive amount of fluid is forced into the subcutaneous tissues, skin necrosis results.

2. Intra-arterial injection: This is a rare complication of IV sedation. Accidental cannulation of an artery should be avoided by good venepuncture technique. Veins should be selected well away from vital structures. The dorsum of the hand is the first choice for venepuncture, because all arteries of that region lie on the ventral surface. If it is necessary to use the antecubital fossa, only superficial veins lateral to the biceps tendon should be used, thereby avoiding the brachial artery and median nerve. All veins should be palpated prior to venepuncture to check for lack of pulsation. At venepuncture the colour of the flashback should be observed, bright red blood indicates that an artery has been penetrated. Intra-arterial cannulation is painful and injection of a test dose of saline will produce discomfort radiating down the arm. At the first sign that an artery may have been entered the injection must be terminated immediately. Pressure should be applied to the site and the arm elevated to prevent the formation of a large haematoma.

The main problem with intra-arterial injection is the potential for subsequent arterial spasm caused by the administration of irritant drugs. Brachial artery spasm is a dangerous condition characterised by an intense burning pain radiating down the arm. The skin blanches and the radial and ulnar pulses weaken to the point of absence. Unless quickly treated the static blood coagulates, causing thrombosis, ischaemia and ultimately gangrene.

Treatment relies on leaving the cannula in place and administering procaine (1%) to promote vasodilatation and to provide local analgesia. The patient should be immediately transferred to hospital where various surgical techniques, the administration of IV heparin or sympathetic blockade may be attempted if the spasm has not resolved. The most widely used sedation agent, midazolam, causes minimal vessel irritation and is unlikely to cause any significant problem if injected into an artery.

3. Post-operative haematoma: Good venepuncture technique is essential to avoid post-operative haematoma and thrombophlebitis. Many patients develop a haematoma at the site of cannulation. This can be prevented by careful venepuncture technique and by ensuring that firm pressure is applied to the puncture wound after removal of the cannula. Poor technique, a damaged cannula, excessively rapid injection or use of an irritant sedation agent, can cause significant vein damage and predispose to thrombophlebitis. The signs of thrombophlebitis can occur from days to weeks after the sedation appointment.

Patients normally present with oedema, inflammation and pain over the course of the vein which was used for cannulation. The infected vein may feel hard and raised. Thrombophlebitis usually improves spontaneously over several weeks. The patient should be kept under review and reassured accordingly until the infection has completely resolved.

4. Injury during sedation and recovery: Finally, sedation patients must be appropriately protected from injury during sedation and recovery. Although sedated patients are conscious, they are less likely to take avoiding action if presented with a noxious stimulus. Protective glasses must be worn by the patient during operative dentistry to prevent dental instruments or materials causing an eye injury. The patient's limbs must be adequately protected from damage caused by equipment such as the bracket table. All electrical equipment must be earthed and no water spray must come into contract with any source of electricity, otherwise there is a risk of electrocution. Naked flames must not be used where oxygen is present as this can cause an explosion.

When patients are moved into the recovery area they must be watched and supported to prevent them from injuring themselves by falling over or hitting sharp objects. It is the responsibility of the dental surgeon to ensure that the sedated patient is protected from accidental injury. Careful instruction must also be given to the escort, who will assume responsibility for the patient from the time of leaving the surgery until full recovery from the effects of the sedation.

References and further reading

British National Formulary. www.bnf.org.

Malamed, S.F. (2000) *Medical Emergencies in the Dental Office.* St Louis, Mosby.

Resuscitation Council (UK) (2005) *Guidelines for Adult Basic Life Support.* London, Resuscitation Council.

Resuscitation Council (UK) (2006) *Medical Emergencies and Resuscitation.* Standards for clinical practice and training for dental practitioners and dental care professionals in general dental practice. London, Resuscitation Council.

Resuscitation Council (UK) (2008) *Emergency Treatment of Anaphylactic Reactions.* Guidelines for healthcare professionals. London, Resuscitation Council.

Resuscitation Council (UK) www.resus.org.uk.

9 Sedation and special care dentistry

INTRODUCTION

Special care dentistry is concerned with providing and enabling the delivery of oral care for people with an impairment or disability, where this terminology is defined in the broadest of terms. Thus, special care dentistry may be considered to be:

'The improvement of oral health of individuals and groups in society, who have a physical, sensory, intellectual, mental, medical, emotional or social impairment or disability or, more often, a combination of a number of these factors.'

The World Health Organization defines disability as an umbrella term, covering impairments, activity limitations and participation restrictions:

'An impairment is a problem in body function or structure; an activity limitation is a difficulty encountered by an individual in executing a task or action; while a participation restriction is a problem experienced by an individual in involvement in life situations. Thus disability is a complex phenomenon, reflecting an interaction between features of a person's body and features of the society in which he or she lives.'

In the UK there are an estimated 11 million adults and 770,000 children with a disability, using the widest survey definition. This equates to more than 1 in 5 adults, and around 1 in 20 children. However, many would not see themselves as disabled, and do not claim disability-related benefits or use services aimed specifically at disabled people.

The population of disabled people includes those with a physical disability, wheelchair users, blind people, deaf people, those with mental health problems and those with medically compromising conditions. Although older people are more likely to be disabled than younger people, trends show an increasing number of children reported as having complex needs, autistic spectrum disorders or mental health issues.

The provision of oral care for disabled people is often complex and time-consuming as a result of their impairment. Additionally, for some people, including those with mental illness and learning disabilities, the issues of informed consent present an added challenge. It is essential to take an holistic approach to oral care to address the complex needs of people in these situations.

Although people with learning disabilities and mental health problems have the same right to equal standards of health and care as the general population, there is evidence that they experience poorer general and oral health, have unmet health needs and have a lower uptake of screening services. The impact of oral conditions on an individual's quality of life can be profound. It has also been reported that oral diseases are less likely to have been treated for people with learning disabilities living in community settings.

Treatment of oral disease is more likely to include extractions rather than fillings, crowns or bridges, particularly for people living in residential care. Physically accessing care for those with disabilities can be problematic. However, another significant barrier is some dentists' attitudes, which can often be negative towards this group of people. There is a need to foster positive attitudes towards disability and to increase the knowledge of those in the dental profession towards disability and oral care.

This chapter will explore the use of conscious sedation in the management of those with disabilities requiring oral health care.

THE USE OF CONSCIOUS SEDATION

Some of the frequently cited reasons for dental neglect in those with disabilities are: inability to locate a dentist willing to perform treatment, financial and transport difficulties, lack of motivation and, most importantly, fear and behavioural problems posed by these patients.

The difficulty in actually carrying out dental treatment may be due to:
• Co-operation, reduced or a complete lack
• Anxiety/phobia
• Exacerbation of a medical condition
• Involuntary movements.

In many cases simple behaviour techniques will enable treatment to be carried out. Where this fails, however, conscious sedation may provide a useful alternative to patient care and avoid the need for general anaesthesia.

In considering management options it is important to consider the following:
- Demand and need for care/long-term plan
- Ease of carrying out treatment
- Different and appropriate options
- Best interests of the patient
- Patient's level of capacity and consent.

The treatment planning process must be realistic and in the best interests of the patient. Management may involve:
- Monitoring and reviewing with no active treatment
- Simple treatment with or without local anaesthesia
- Treatment with conscious sedation and local anaesthesia
- Treatment under general anaesthetic.

The final decision to use conscious sedation must involve:
- Consultation with the patient and/or carer
- Assessment of medical and social history and fitness
- Consent process
- Most appropriate location for treatment.

The provision of conscious sedation in special care dentistry will be presented under the following headings:
1. Location for providing conscious sedation
2. Patient groups:
    - Neurological disorders
    - Musculoskeletal disorders
    - Learning disability
    - Sensory disability
    - Mental health problems
    - Systemic conditions (see Chapter 3).

Location for providing conscious sedation

For conscious sedation to be safe, valuable and effective, it is essential that the most appropriate type of conscious sedation is chosen for each individual and administered in the correct environment by an appropriately trained practitioner. Conscious sedation for dental care may be provided in two different settings:

Out-patient setting

- General dental practice
- Community dental practice
- Dental hospital setting.

Day-stay setting

- Anaesthetist led hospital unit.

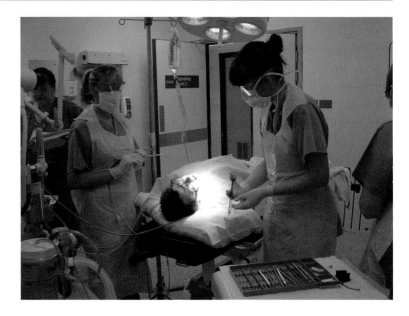

The main criterion used to determine the most appropriate
setting for patient care is the ASA grade. Patients classified as
ASA I and II can generally be managed on an out-patient basis
under intravenous sedation or inhalation sedation. Some ASA
III patients can be managed with inhalation sedation in this
setting.

Patients classified as ASA III requiring intravenous
sedation, who present a greater risk, should be managed in
an anaesthetist-led, hospital day-stay setting, where back-up
facilities are readily available and extended recovery is possible
where required (Figure 9.1). The day-stay facility will also allow
for medical investigations to be carried out if required. Very
rarely do patients require management on an in-patient basis,
although there may be some exceptions to this.

When providing dental care for people with disabilities the
practitioner must be fully competent in the management of the
individual's condition. More often than not the actual dental
treatment itself is simple, complicated only by the effects of
the disability. Referral of such patients to clinicians with the
appropriate experience and knowledge in the field of special
care dentistry, may be necessary to ensure the patient receives
the most effective care.

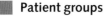 **Patient groups**

 Neurological conditions

The presence of a neurological impairment can be a major
barrier to the receipt of oral care, both in accessing the service

and in being able to receive dental treatment. The ability to receive dental treatment relies on patients being able to sit in the dental chair, open their mouth and allow procedures to be carried out. This is not always possible for those who are restricted physically or who present with involuntary muscle co-ordination. Examples of such conditions include:

- Multiple sclerosis
- Parkinson's disease
- Cerebral palsy
- Stroke
- Huntington's disease.

Many of these patients are also anxious about the effect their disability might have on them receiving care. The management of such patients can be assisted by the use of conscious sedation. As well as the anxiolytic effect, one of the main benefits lies in the muscle relaxation achieved by the sedative technique, in particular the use of intravenous midazolam.

Involuntary movements are a feature of cerebral palsy, Parkinson's disease, multiple sclerosis and Huntington's disease and greatly hinder the provision of oral care. Providing muscle relaxation by way of conscious sedation is of great benefit to patients and clinicians. It is important to be aware that many patients may have an impaired swallowing ability as a result of their condition and when providing treatment under conscious sedation the patient should be kept in the semi-prone position. It is essential to have a high power suction unit to ensure the airway is kept clear at all times.

As well as the main neurological features of these conditions, some patients will present with other problems including learning disability, dementia and associated medical conditions. It is therefore essential to carry out a full medical and social assessment prior to agreeing the most appropriate management option.

Musculoskeletal disorders

Musculoskeletal disorders are those affecting the bones, joints, cartilage, tendons, ligaments and muscles. The severity of the condition can range from mild transitory conditions to more severe disabling effects.

The main difficulty in maintaining and receiving oral care is the inability physically to carry out basic oral hygiene, to access the dental surgery and to sit comfortably in the dental chair and allow oral access. Some of the more common disorders include arthritis, ankylosing spondylitis, and congenital and genetic disorders.

A combination of the muscle relaxant and anxiolytic effects of sedative drugs can help to reduce muscle spasm, improving access to the oral cavity and increasing the general comfort for the patient.

Very often however, venous access can be difficult in these patients owing to arthritic hand and finger joints, and if intravenous sedation is indicated it is imperative to ensure the clinician/sedationist has relevant experience in managing such cases.

Learning disability

The term learning disability can be defined as 'a significant impairment of intelligence and social functioning acquired before adulthood'. Examples of specific conditions include:

- Autism
- Down syndrome
- Attention deficit and hyperactivity disorder (ADHD)
- Cerebral palsy
- Other congenital or genetic disorders.

Many individuals with these conditions may have associated disability including physical, sensory or medical impairments. The main problem delivering care to those with a learning disability lies in the patient's level of co-operation and understanding. Learning disabilities range in severity and often are described as mild, moderate or severe. This classification can be linked to intellectual ability and IQ; those with a lower IQ having a more profound learning disability. In addition to IQ and intellectual ability, it is also essential to understand the impact a person's disability has on his or her life.

Conscious sedation may be indicated in those patients with a mild learning disability who have some difficulty in co-operating for dental care, but who are able to sit in the dental chair. The patient must have a degree of understanding such that they appreciate how the sedation can help them. Without this basic understanding, many patients become confused and disorientated, leading to agitation and limited co-operation.

As with all patients, a thorough medical and social history is required, to assess fitness for sedation and dental treatment and to ensure the treatment is provided in the most appropriate setting.

Sensory impairment

Sensory impairments include hearing and visual impairments. The impairments themselves rarely create a direct problem with the delivery of dental care, however many patients with such impairments may be increasingly anxious about attending the dental surgery and the inherent problems this may hold for them.

Hearing impairment can range from mild to profound hearing loss or deafness and people will communicate in a variety of ways by use of sign language, lip reading, hearing aids and body language.

A patient who is sedated will be less alert and communicative and this situation will be compounded for those with a hearing impairment. It is therefore essential to discuss the complete treatment plan, methods of treatment and sedative effects with the patient before commencing treatment. The use of inhalation sedation may not be indicated as the technique relies on hypnotic suggestion, which would be difficult to achieve in patients with hearing difficulties.

Visual impairment may not cause as many difficulties but excellent communication skills are required to keep the patient informed at all stages.

Mental health problems

The term 'mental health problem' covers a wide range of issues which affect someone's ability to get on with their daily life. Mental health problems can affect anyone, of any age and background, and have an impact on family, friends and carers. On average 1 in 4 people will experience some kind of mental health problem in the course of a year. However, of these, only a relatively small number will be diagnosed with a serious and enduring condition. The mental health problem may be mild, causing emotional distress which is transitory or may be more severe, interfering with the person's ability to cope on a day-to-day basis.

Mental health problems include:
- Neuroses
  - Anxiety states
  - Depression
  - Obsessive compulsive disorder (OCD)
  - Post-traumatic stress disorder (PTSD)
- Psychoses
  - Bipolar disorder
  - Psychotic depression
  - Delirium
  - Dementia
  - Schizophrenia
  - Substance abuse
- Psychosomatic disorders

- Anorexia and bulimia
- Personality disorders.

People with mental health problems can experience anxiety about dental care which may be compounded by their condition. The use of conscious sedation to help alleviate stress and anxiety during care can therefore be extremely valuable. The provision of sedation for those with mental health problems may be influenced by the level and stability of the patient's condition, the type of medication the patient may be taking, and the patient's level of mental capacity.

A patient who has a mild or well-controlled mental health disorder, for example mild depression or well-controlled schizophrenia, will benefit from inhalation or intravenous sedation. In the majority of cases these patients can be treated in a primary care setting.

In more severe cases, where the patient's level of understanding and co-operation is perhaps altered, their condition is poorly controlled or where the individual is on a multiple drug regimen, an anaesthetist-led, hospital day-stay service may be more suitable. Managing such patients on a day-stay basis allows for closer monitoring over a longer period of time. Premedication can be easily administered, should this be felt necessary, to help the patient cope with the sedation technique and subsequent treatment. In the event of an untoward incident, emergency care is readily available.

The deciding factor for location of treatment will rest with the patient's ASA classification, which depends on the severity of their disability and any concomitant systemic conditions. It is also important to consider drug interactions; many of the drugs used in the treatment of mental health conditions are central nervous system depressants and can produce a synergistic effect when combined with benzodiazepines used for conscious sedation. The opposite is also true, whereby some patients may build up a tolerance to sedative agents, leading to an ineffective technique. Patients who are recreational drug users present a similar dilemma.

SUMMARY

The provision of oral care to people with disabilities can be greatly enhanced using conscious sedation. The choice of technique should be the simplest and safest form available for a particular individual carried out in an appropriate setting.

A variety of sedation techniques, for this group of patients, have been reported in the literature in cluding intravenous, oral, transmucosal and inhalation. The decision on the most suitable option should only be made following a thorough assessment of the patient's cognitive function, level of cooperation, physical ability, medical history and social cirumstances.

References and further reading

British Institute for Learning Disabilities: www.bild.org.

British Society for Disability and Oral Health (2001) *Clinical Guidelines and Integrated Care Pathways for the Oral Health Care of People with Learning Disabilities.* Oxford, British Society for Disability and Oral Health.

Griffiths, J. & Boyle, S. (2005) *Holistic Oral Care. A Guide for Health Professionals.* London, Stephen Hancocks Limited: p. 249.

Joint Advisory Committee for Special Care Dentistry (2003) *A Case for Need: Proposal for a Specialty in Special Care Dentistry.* Oxford, British Society for Disability and Oral Health.

Lawton, L. (2002) Providing dental care for special patients: tips for the general dentist. *Journal of the American Dental Association*, **133**(12), 1666–1670.

Locker, D. (1992) The burden of oral disorders in populations of older adults. *Community Dental Health*, **9**(2), 109–124.

Manley, M. C., Ransford, N. J., Lewis, D. A., Thompson, S. A., Forbes, M. (2008) Retrospective audit of the efficacy and safety of the combined intranasal/intravenous sedation technique for the dental treatment of adults with learning disability. *British Dental Journal*, **205**(2): E3; discussion 84–5. Epub 2008 June 13.

Manley, M.C., Skelly, A.M. & Hamilton, A.G. (2000) Dental treatment for people with challenging behaviour: general anaesthesia or sedation? *British Dental Journal*, **188**(7), 358–360.

Mental Health Foundation: www.mentalhealth.org.uk.

Prime Minister's Strategy Unit (2005) *Improving the Life Chances of Disabled People. Final Report.* London, Strategy Unit Disability Team.

Tiller, S., Wilson, K.I. & Gallagher, J.E. (2001) Oral health status and dental service use of adults with learning disabilities living in residential institutions and in the community. *Community Dental Health*, **18**(3), 167–171.

World Health Organization (2008) Disabilities. Available: www.who.int/topics/disabilities/en. Accessed 15 August 2008.

10 Medico-legal and ethical considerations

INTRODUCTION

This chapter introduces some of the medico-legal and ethical issues that surround sedation and the practice of dentistry. It is impossible to cover the subject in its entirety and for more detailed information the reader is advised to search the medico-legal literature. Medico-legal issues are a necessity of into modern clinical practice. It is essential that clinicians practising sedation have a good understanding of medico-legal issues relating to clinical practice; the basic principles will be addressed in the following chapter.

THE LEGAL SYSTEM IN THE UK

There are two parallel legal systems in Britain – the criminal system and the civil system.

Criminal system

In the criminal system, charges are usually heard in the magistrates and crown courts and the issue at stake is on the question of guilt. The choice of court is usually dependent on the seriousness of the charge and prosecutions may start in a lower court before being transferred to a higher court.

Civil system

In civil cases the question concerned is of injury to a person or his/her property and the issue to be determined is whether or not compensation should be paid. Cases will be heard by a judge or registrar (a junior judge) and there will be no jury present. In the civil system, small claims are usually heard in the county courts whilst the High Courts oversee all the lower courts.

Dentists face the possibility of actions in either the criminal or the civil systems. There are fundamental differences between the courts and the ways they work and there are differences within the United Kingdom, particularly in Scotland which has its own judicial system. As implied earlier, one of the principal differences is on the question of guilt. In the criminal courts, the concept of guilt is absolute; a person is either guilty or not guilty and will be judged and punished accordingly. Mitigating factors may be taken into account but in general terms these relate to the circumstances surrounding a situation rather than the details of the crime itself.

In the civil courts decisions are based on the 'balance of probability' and compensation is determined accordingly. There are appeal systems for both the criminal and civil courts, referred to as the Court of Appeal, although it is actually comprised of two distinct courts. In neither case are witnesses called but rather legal arguments are put forward as to why the original decision was wrong. Finally, appeals against the decisions of the Court of Appeal can be made to the House of Lords although this process has to be applied for (or 'leave given') and these appeals are usually only allowed on contentious issues.

Clinical staff are well advised to understand the basic principles of law and how they may be affected by any charges brought against them. In this regard, both patient and dentist have certain rights and responsibilities and these are considered below. The European Court of Justice also has a duty to oversee the legal structures of member countries to ensure that the law is being applied fairly in member states. In other countries, legal systems vary considerably and the differing ways of administering the law can have a profound effect on the way justice is determined.

RIGHTS AND RESPONSIBILITIES OF A PATIENT

The primary and fundamental rights of all patients relate first to the principle of self-determination (autonomy) and second to the expectation that any medical or surgical intervention offered should, above all else, safeguard the health of the recipient. In general terms, this means that the benefit of any procedure should substantially outweigh any associated risks. In extreme cases, for example where a potentially life saving operation may carry a high risk of mortality, the patient should be made aware of the consequences of intervening or not intervening. In essence, this is the basis on which the principle of consent operates and this is explained more fully below. It requires that all health professionals always put the patient's interests first and that they do not let themselves become unduly influenced by their own personal preferences. (A classic example where this approach sometimes is seen to be lacking is on oncology clinics, when the views of radiotherapists and surgeons on the treatment of cancer frequently appear divergent and not always related to best known clinical practice.) It is important to consider the following patient expectations:

Patient's best interests

With the requirements for sedation, the patient's best interests must be served by any decision to recommend or withhold the offer of sedation. In this regard the concept of the 'sedation practice', where everybody has sedation all the time, is not a good one. It is self-evident that any patient who does not require sedation for a particular procedure should not have it offered or administered.

Expert advice

Patients also have the right to expect expert advice. Because of the privileged nature of the dental profession and its protected status in law, patients must be given appropriate, accurate and current information regarding any condition they have or treatment they are to receive. This can only be achieved by practitioners keeping up to date with modern developments through education and self-improvement. Where a dentist is unable to provide accurate details on a relevant subject the information should be obtained from a third party.

Quality care

This combination of expert advice based on safeguarding the patient's health as a primary responsibility, should automatically lead to the third area of expectation – the receipt of quality care. Quality care is difficult to define but readily understandable. It is the prospect of having treatment which will be both effective and durable. There can be little doubt that the majority of all dental treatment performed in this country fits the above criteria but there are times when this is not the case. On occasion this may be due to inadequate treatment or failed materials and sometimes it is due to mistakes being made.

The law does not deny the likelihood of mistakes occurring but it does expect mistakes to be corrected, and patients can expect the support of the law in this regard. The question as to whether a 'mistake' is of such severity that it would be considered negligent is not the same issue. The primary question in law to be answered first is whether the practitioner making the mistake was using reasonable skill when the accident occurred, and second, was the opportunity given to remedy the error. Many cases have been lost by plaintiffs on this latter point.

Plaintiffs in negligence cases also have a duty to submit themselves for examination by an expert witness for the defence, if required so to do. This is supposed to prevent the malicious pursuit of a claim against a practitioner when, if such access was not agreed, the patient could effectively frustrate a reasonable defence. The same principle would apply to any medical records held on behalf of a patient which may relate to an incident and these can be requested by the defendant or the plaintiff.

DUTIES AND RESPONSIBILITIES OF THE DENTIST

Direct patient care

The converse of the above section clearly applies. In delivering care to a patient the dentist must safeguard:
- The patient's health
- Provide the patient with expert information
- Deliver quality care
- Remedy any mistakes which may occur.

A dentist does not have to conform to a single opinion with reference to a particular technique, method or procedure. There may even be disagreements on the matter of diagnosis and again this possibility is recognised by the courts. The law provides specific protection in this regard and the test applied is known as the 'Bolam Principle' which is that;

'One cannot be guilty of negligence providing that the action is one which is in accordance with a practice accepted as proper by a responsible body of (medical/dental) opinion even though another body of opinion may take a contrary view'.

With reference to the degree of skill required by the practitioner, the test is the 'standard of the ordinary skilled man exercising and professing to have that particular skill'. This level of skill is effectively defined by the body of opinion of the particular specialty. (In Ireland the situation is slightly complicated because the plaintiff could still prove liability on the part of the dentist if it could be shown that despite a practice being accepted it had obvious and inherent defects, and a recent case in Britain has adopted a similar view.) It would be true to say, however, that the majority of medico-legal problems today are associated with issues relating to negligence and the question of consent.

The dentist has an absolute duty to obtain the consent of a patient before undertaking any procedure. Failure to do so may constitute assault and battery although, in reality, charges of this nature are usually rejected by the courts in favour of negligence claims. The question of consent is extensive and is dealt with later in this chapter.

Record keeping

In addition to the legal constraints outlined above, the dentist also has other duties that would reasonably be expected of a professional. These include, for example, keeping good, accurate and contemporaneous records. This is a common area of inadequacy and one which is frequently compounded by the retrospective addition of notes when problems occur. These are normally added in an attempt to clarify details but they have little standing in law and can make the defence of a case untenable. Notes must, therefore, be made as contemporaneously as possible but never to the detriment of clinical practice.

The notes made by a dentist and all the other information gathered about patients is confidential and there are very few occasions when it can be legally disclosed without the patient's consent. The right of confidentiality is well understood in law and can only be breached in well-defined circumstances. Dental records must therefore be kept promptly, accurately and confidentially.

Legal and professional restraints

The final area of responsibility of a dentist is that of observing legal and professional restraints. The law may influence clinical practice in a variety of ways, some obvious and some remote. The law exists to protect the patient and its influence is profound, perhaps no more so than in the Dental Act which gives statutory powers to the General Dental Council (GDC). In other countries other regulatory bodies exist with varying degrees of power. In the UK, however, the GDC issues professional guidance and with regard to sedation its recommendations are quite specific. The dentist has a duty to observe the guidance given by the council and failure to do so may result in a charge of professional misconduct and the dentist will have to provide answer to any such charges. On a more positive note, however, the GDC provides professional

recognition for the dentist and it has enormous powers to stop
the misappropriate use of dentistry.

Further restraints and guidance can be imposed by many
authorities including the fire services, the Health and Safety
Executive, etc. It behoves each member of the dental practice to
be aware of the prevailing conditions and to pay due attention
to their requirements.

CRIMINAL AND CIVIL CHARGES

The terms assault and battery are frequently used and poorly
understood. Assault is technically the threat of violence against
a person rather than the act of violence itself. Battery may be
defined as any unwarranted physical contact but usually refers
to an act that violates somebody. A person cannot be guilty
of battery if he/she can prove that the contact was entirely
accidental or that he/she was acting with the person's
agreement. In some medico-legal cases some plaintiffs have
tried to bring criminal proceedings, claiming assault and
battery based on technical questions of consent, but this has
rarely been successful. The courts have usually decreed that
claims for medical accidents should be heard under charges of
negligence, i.e. as a civil claim rather than a criminal offence.

This may have some advantages, but for a patient, it does
mean that until they go to court and successfully prove that
negligence has occurred, it is impossible to know whether
they are entitled to any compensation. To successfully prove
negligence, a plaintiff must show:
1. that a duty of care was owed
2. that the duty of care was breached
3. that the breach in care resulted in harm to the patient.

Patients usually have no problem in proving the duty of care
was owed but to simultaneously prove points 2 and 3 above is
not always easy. This sometimes leads to decisions which, to
say the least, seem arbitrary.

In some cases the question of negligence is highly
controversial and the court system is both expensive and
unpredictable. Because of this there has been a considerable
amount of criticism of the litigation system, and in some
countries 'no-fault' compensation schemes exist for medical
accidents, where compensation is awarded on fixed scales
of payments but where the plaintiff does not have to prove
negligence after a medical accident to get compensation. It
could be argued that such a scheme is preferable, although
there are also opponents to such systems who argue that it
could lower professional standards.

▇▇▇▇ CONSENT

Patients have a fundamental legal and ethical right to determine what happens to their own bodies. Valid consent to treatment is therefore absolutely central in all forms of health care, from providing personal care to undertaking major surgery.

Consent in the medical context is a patient's agreement for a health professional to provide care. Patients may indicate consent non-verbally (for example by presenting their arm for their pulse to be taken), orally, or in writing. For the consent to be valid, the patient must:

- be competent to take the particular decision
- have received sufficient information to take it
- not be acting under duress.

A person may choose without undue pressure to give or withhold consent to any examination, investigation or treatment as a matter of choice. If a patient has given his or her consent to a procedure being undertaken, there can be no grounds for bringing a charge of battery (although they may still be able to claim the breach of negligence). In a court of law, therefore, the issue is simply one of whether a patient had consented, and the practitioner has to be able to demonstrate that this was the case.

▇▇▇▇ Demonstrating consent

In some cases this may be possible simply by referring to the actions of the patient, for example, lying in a dental chair and opening one's mouth is almost certainly sufficient evidence of a patient consenting to an oral examination. No written signature is necessary in such cases but conversely, a signature obtained on an illegible consent form is unlikely to be acceptable evidence of consent in complex restoration cases carried out under intravenous sedation. This is because the dentist has a duty of care to the patient to explain, in such a way that the patient understands the nature of the procedure being proposed, its associated risks and benefits and any possible alternative treatments. Modern consent forms nearly always include a section which is signed by practitioners certifying that they have explained the details to the patient. Even so, it should be remembered that the consent form in itself is not necessarily sufficient evidence of consent being obtained.

▇▇▇▇ Patient information

There is also the question of how much information should be given, and this is not defined in law. Two classic cases are often quoted in the legal literature with reference to this: the Sidaway case and the Bolam case.

Returning to the latter case again, Mr Bolam was given electroconvulsive therapy (ECT) to treat depression. As a result he sustained two fractures and sued his doctor for negligence, especially as the doctor was aware of the risks and failed to warn him. The judge found in favour of the defendant, arguing that the doctor had complied with accepted medical opinion and that for Mr Bolam to succeed in his action he would have had to show that he would not have proceeded with treatment had he been made aware of the risks of treatment.

In Mrs Sidaway's case, she was tragically paralysed by surgery to her back, but again judgement went against her claim against the surgeon because the degree of risk was low and a body of neurosurgeons would not have routinely warned patients of the possibility of paralysis.

In defining how much information a patient should be given, this judgement sets out the principle that it should be enough for the patient to make an informed decision. It is, therefore, probably not necessary to warn every patient that there is a small fraction of a chance of dying from sedation but it is probably negligent to fail to warn a patient of a possible numb lip after surgically removing a deeply impacted second premolar.

Patient age

The question of a person's age is also relevant to the laws of consent. The law defines adulthood from the date of a person's eighteenth birthday. From that age, providing they have the capacity to make decisions on their own behalf, people are said to be competent. To be deemed competent, an adult must be able to:

- understand the proposed treatment in relation to its benefits and risks
- understand the alternative treatments available
- understand the consequences of not accepting the proposed treatment
- retain the relevant information long enough to make a free decision, i.e. with no external pressure from any interested party.

The law is complicated for children between the ages of 16 and 18 years and even more so for those under 16 years. In essence, however, the same general principles hold true for children when they consent (agree) to treatment. In the past, it has been traditional to ask parents to sign consent on behalf of their children under the age of sixteen but, in law, children may now legally sign consent for both surgery and sedation if they are

competent to do so. The age at which they become competent
is not defined but it can no longer be set rigidly at age 16. If
children refuse to consent to treatment, however, their parents
may well have a legal right to overrule their refusal. This is
unquestionably so with young children but must be exercised
with progressive caution as children get older. The same rights
can be given to the courts in making a child a Ward of Court but
such actions need to be taken with some sensitivity. Consent
may also be given by legal guardians, adoptive parents and the
local authorities for children who are the subject of a care order.

Capacity to consent

Finally, the hardest area in the question of consent is probably
in relation to those adult patients who are not deemed
competent. At the current time nobody can authorise consent
on behalf of an incompetent adult (except in cases where they
have predetermined it by an advanced power of attorney) and
doctors and dentists must act in their patient's best interests,
wherever possible obtaining two independent professional
views as to the advisability of any proposed treatment. A record
should be made of the assessment of the patient's capacity,
why the health professional believes the treatment to be in the
patient's best interests, and the involvement of people close to
the patient.

The practitioner's overriding responsibility is the duty of
care which is owed to the patient and, if necessary, this should
be demonstrable to a court of law. Parents may give consent
on behalf of children between the ages of 16 and 18 years when
the child is not deemed competent to do so. The law on these
matters has recently changed as a result of the 2005 Mental
Capacity Act (England and Wales) and expert opinion should
be sought in any case likely to be contentious.

Assessing capacity to give consent

The Mental Capacity Act for England and Wales (2005) in
dealing with the issue of capacity states that:
- A person must be assumed to have capacity unless it is
established that he lacks capacity
- A person is not to be treated as unable to make a decision
unless all practicable steps to help him to do so have been
taken without success
- A person is not to be treated as unable to make a decision
merely because he makes an unwise decision
- An act done or decision made, under this Act for or on behalf
of a person who lacks capacity must be done, or made, in his
best interests

- Before the act is done, or the decision is made, regard must be had to whether the purpose for which it is needed can be as effectively achieved in a way that is less restrictive of the person's rights and freedom of action.

In assessing a person's capacity the following factors must be met:
- Can the patient understand and retain the relevant treatment information?
- Does the patient believe it?
- Can the patient weigh the information in the balance to arrive at a choice?

If the patient fails to meet any of these tests he or she will lack capacity and the clinician treating the patient can act in the best interests of the patient.

The situation in Scotland differs in that, where an adult lacks capacity to consent (other than in an emergency, or where there is a proxy decision maker), a certificate of incapacity must be issued to provide care or treatment.

RISK ASSESSMENT

Risk assessment is essentially a management tool, used to minimise the incidence of untoward events, but it can be applied to clinical situations with great effect. It is a process which should be proactive and not reactive, i.e. it should attempt to stop mistakes before they happen rather than using the mistakes themselves as the drivers of change.

Areas to be considered in a risk assessment include information and consent, staff training issues, referral mechanism, standardised procedures, and standard facilities, amongst others. Risk assessment should be dealt with systematically and repeated periodically. Any problems identified should be addressed and solutions put in place which should themselves be assessed after a period of time. All staff members must be included in the process and encouraged to strive for continued improvement in standards.

DEALING WITH SEDATION-RELATED INCIDENTS

The incidence of complications from patients undergoing simple sedation for dental treatment is extremely low. However, there have been reports of critical episodes, some of which have led to serious morbidity. In such cases there will be a sequence of procedures to be followed and questions to be asked. The purpose of this is to establish:

1. What went wrong and why did it go wrong?
2. Had a proper pre-assessment procedure been followed?
3. Was the sedation technique used justifiable and correctly administered by a competent person?
4. Were the appropriate support staff available at all times?
5. Was a correct resuscitation procedure followed by staff who knew and performed their duties, and were all the necessary drugs and equipment available?

If the dentist can give reasons, for the first question and answer the remaining questions positively, there will be little cause for concern. If not, the failings need to be identified so that the courts can determine a verdict in relation to the adverse event.

Everyone concerned with the practice of sedation must ensure that it is a safe, efficient and effective procedure which is undertaken for the benefit of the patient. In the vast majority of cases this will be beyond doubt; in the few cases where mishaps occur, careful and prompt management should ensure that a minor problem does not become a clinical or a legal catastrophe. For most patients, conscious sedation enables them to undertake dental treatment which they would at best find uncomfortable and at worst, impossible. For the dentist, it offers a set of tools which can aid in treatment provision and general patient management.

References and further reading

Department of Health (2001) *Good Practice in Consent Implementation Guide: Consent to Examination or Treatment.* London, HMSO.

Johnston, C. & Liddle, J. (2007) The Mental Capacity Act 2005: a new framework for healthcare decision making. *Journal of Medical Ethics*, **33**(2), 94–97.

Mental Capacity Act 2005. Available: www.opsi.gov.uk/ACTS/acts2005/ukpga_20050009_en_1. Accessed 18 August 2008.

Scottish Government (2000) Adults with Incapacity (Scotland) Act 2000.

Index

Page numbers in *italics* represent figures, those in **bold** represent tables.